WITHDRAWN

The Food Nanny

The Ten Food Rules to prevent a frighteningly fat future for your kids

WITHDRAWN

WITHDRAWN

KILKENNY COUNTY LIBRARY

KK424649

About the Author

Having graduated from Trinity College Dublin with a degree in microbiology, and University College Cork in 1995 with a master's degree in nutrition, Anna Burns has amassed over seventeen years' experience in the field of nutrition. With experience ranging from working in New Zealand's food supplement industry to living and working in France, Anna returned to Ireland in 1999 to work in health promotion with the Irish Health Board. She now runs her nutrition consultancy from Cork and delivers corporate nutrition training countrywide. She runs two weight-loss clinics in Cork and has a 'no gimmicks' approach to fat loss.

Anna currently lives in Cork with her husband and four children, who have, unwittingly, been her subjects for testing her old-fashioned approach to healthy eating for years.

Praise for Anna Burns

'Thanks to Anna's programme I learned how to understand the food I eat and how my body works with this food. Anna has taught me which foods encourage a healthier lifestyle and healthier living – all with a no-nonsense, practical approach to eating food which is healthy, nutritious, tasty and satisfying.'

Breda, Limerick

'I was absolutely blown away by Anna's knowledge and, in particular, her unique and witty style of delivery. I can safely say our family's eating habits have improved and changed for the better.'

Michael, Cork

'Anna gave a talk to parents at our primary school. Her session was captivating and very relevant to us all. Her influence on my family's food habits has led to a shift in thinking when it comes to food choices that my children now make and a shift in lifestyle for us in general.'

Paula, Cork

'I can finally stop dieting now that Anna has taught me how to balance my diet. I am grateful that I will be able to teach my children a balanced way to eat and not worry about "right" and "wrong" foods any more.'

Margaret, Cork

'My family eats what I eat now, vegetables and all, which is something I never thought would happen.'
Linda, Cork

'With the tools Anna's approach has given me, I am now looking forward to my daughter growing into her current weight and never concerning herself with dieting. Without even meeting her, Anna has changed my daughter's life!'
Mary, Cork

'Over the ten-week period of consulting Anna my family's life has changed beyond recognition. Gone are the crisps and weekly takeaway. Now I cook every meal from scratch. I don't spend hours in the kitchen, I cook simple and tasty foods and I shop to a plan. Anna delivered on all of her promises!'
Grace, Cork

The Food Nanny

The Ten Food Rules to prevent a
frighteningly fat future for your kids

Anna Burns

KILKENNY
COUNTY
LIBRARY

Gill & Macmillan

Accession No: KK424649
Price: EUR10.49
55548
THE BOOK NEST LTD
130710

Gill & Macmillan
Hume Avenue, Park West
Dublin 12
with associated companies throughout the world
www.gillmacmillanbooks.ie

© Anna Burns 2012

ISBN: 978 07171 5471 5

Print origination by TypeIT, Dublin
Indexed by Róisín Nic Cóil
Printed and bound by CPI Group (UK) Ltd, Croydon, CR0 4YY

This book is typeset in 10pt Minion.
The paper used in this book comes from the wood pulp of managed
forests. For every tree felled, at least one tree is planted, thereby
renewing natural resources.
All rights reserved. No part of this publication may be copied,
reproduced or transmitted in any form or by any means, without
permission of the publisher.
A catalogue record for this book is available from the British Library.

5 4 3 2 1

Contents

	Introduction	1
Rule 1:	I can say 'No' to food	13
Rule 2:	Eat only at the table	31
Rule 3:	Have they had their fruit and vegetables today?	49
Rule 4:	We do not need to buy organic foods	77
Rule 5:	If you can name it, you can consider it	99
Rule 6:	Say 'No' to passive consumption	123
Rule 7:	Eat only when you feel hungry	143
Rule 8:	Get moving!	165
Rule 9:	Just portion control it	183
Rule 10:	Have a strategy	201
	Forward to a fun, fit future	223
	Index	233

This book is dedicated to my husband, Tom.
With appreciation for my parents, a direct link with a more formal era.
And a big thank you to my sources of inspiration: Ciara, Louis, Hannah and William.
A sincere thank you also to Nicki and everyone at Gill & Macmillan.
And a final word of thanks to my sister, Sheila, for her ongoing support.

Introduction

We have lost our way when it comes to balanced nutrition for the entire family, whether for reasons of business, distraction, advertising, the media, lack of discipline or a combination of these. Good food is often perceived to be expensive and time-consuming to prepare: perhaps even complicated, involving convoluted recipes. Because of our desire for quick-fix meal solutions and instant gratification, we are breeding a generation of potentially overweight kids with no appreciation for the simple tastes of non-processed foods. This is more apparent in Ireland and Britain than it is elsewhere in Europe: we are the fattest of them all. Our obesity levels are constantly on the rise and our kids are getting dangerously fat.

We are all aware of how serious the situation currently is in North America. You only have to watch any American reality show to get a feel for how scary the future must be for many American kids. Until the 1990s I had never seen more than the very occasional obese child or teenager. Up to that point in our history most of our kids – in Ireland and Britain – were of an appropriate size, and only the occasional child tended towards overweight. Today this has all changed. If we follow the American experience, we will be looking down the barrel of a very fat future for our children, who will become obese adults and who will live shorter than expected lives. Our kids' generation may, as is the American situation today, be the first in the history of our evolution not to outlive their parents.

This is not (yet) the case in many other European countries. The populations of countries such as France, Switzerland, Italy, Norway and Sweden still have low levels of obesity. They also consume more fruit and vegetables than other European countries (no surprise there). Having lived and worked in France I can attest to this fact. French people eat lots and lots of salad and green vegetables. They do not eat between meals. They never eat 'diet' foods. They drink moderate amounts of alcohol and they have 'to-die-for' desserts. They even smoke! And yet they do not die as young as we do! Recently, though, obesity levels have doubled in France, as they have in other countries, so the traditional approach to eating might be slipping somewhat for the French too. That said, they still have among the lowest obesity levels in Europe.

When I was completing my master's degree in nutrition I worked as a laboratory assistant at l'Institut Nationale de la Recherche Agronomique (INRA) in Nantes on the western coast of France, exploring the physical and chemical properties of pea and apple fibre. What amazed me then (1993) was that in an industrial area outside the beautiful city of Nantes one could have a two-hour lunch break with nothing to do other than eat and chat. The concept of a leisurely lunch, while at work, with nothing to distract from the potential boredom of it all, was alien to me. I learned a lot that summer, not necessarily about pea and apple fibre, but about balance and good habits around food. The staff (mainly highly qualified researchers) were so lovely and welcoming that I would spend these two hours every day, five days a week, chatting, observing and then emulating their eating habits. I could never bring myself to order a little glass of wine at lunch as so many others did, though – I wouldn't have had a hope of going back to the lab after lunchtime to meticulously record minute details of an ongoing experiment! I do remember, however, changing how I ate that summer. One thing I instantly noticed was how long it took to eat the many courses that constituted lunch. First might come sausages on lentils, which would be eaten with a little bread; ten minutes later there might be a simple green salad, in splendid isolation; another twenty minutes might pass before a plain yoghurt would be eaten, with maybe half a sachet of sugar stirred into it; and finally a pear might appear, of which half would be eaten, the other half left on the plate. Before I went to France, my lunch would have been the likes of a ham sandwich and packet of crisps, eaten in about fifteen minutes flat!

Today I holiday with my family in France every summer. We eat fresh white peaches from the market during August; we get the best bread imaginable every day from the local bakery; we drink wine; we eat al fresco every day – and we eat more McDonald's during that trip than for the rest of the year put together. I do not lie! Today, the French love McDonald's. You will find 'Macdo' in every town, off every stretch of motorway, and this is why, while travelling down through France at the start of our holidays and on the return journey, we will stop off to give the kids a break in the magical Old McDonald's (as my four-year-old calls it) play zone and have our lunch. Ironic, isn't it? My kids associate France with eating McDonald's!

The reality is that traditional eating habits have begun to move out of the grasp of many busy working – or unemployed – families in France, as they have in much of the rest of Europe. While the French will, no doubt, keep on top of this trend by making policy and working hard to maintain their way of life, we have no such strong basis on which to call. We are not known world-wide for our fabulous food or for the variety and colour of our fresh produce. We look back to times when we ate frugally – times of food rationing in the World War II era, for instance – as times of hardship, even of famine. What we should remember is that in this current time of abundance, of affordable food, our issue is now one of restraint. **We need, in fact, to go back to old-fashioned eating, to a style that our parents or grandparents followed.** We can also emulate the traditional French way of eating, which is still very much apparent among most French adults. The scene in my work canteen, for example, was only twenty years ago. While today fewer workplaces offer a two-hour lunch break, most French organisations still produce well-balanced meals with just as many courses.

The reason I began to write this book is that in my weight-loss business, it struck me repeatedly that the poor habits demonstrated by many of us as adults, which have led us to become overweight, have also become the norm for our kids. This translates into a frighteningly fat future for our kids, a future of overweight and of constant dieting. We need to correct this situation now, and we really can once we know what to do and how to approach it. It is never too late for anyone to start on their journey to a healthy weight; and it is not too late for your kids.

As I iron out my clients' eating habits, I teach them the basic rules of good dietary habits. These include such rules as always sitting down to eat; following a plan for weekly food shopping; eating out without overdoing it; and reading food labels effectively. When we discuss such plans, parents often also enquire about their children's diets with a view to improving them. **In all cases I tell parents that children learn through the example set by parents' own improved habits.** In my corporate work – when I talk to large groups in the workplace setting, for instance – I find that many parents are concerned that their kids eat too many of the wrong foods, are picky eaters or are overweight. Should they regularly be allowed to eat ice cream, fast foods or sweets? How can they come to like their most hated vegetables? These and similar questions usually emerge from those talks.

I am not advocating spending hours in the kitchen, making your own bread, scrubbing and peeling every evening. No. For the most part I tend to buy my potatoes washed and with a skin I am happy to eat; that's two jobs done! We have to simplify our expectations of what good food looks and tastes like. Of course our children will love oven chips with sausages if that's what they always get. They are designed to love salt and fat. For reasons of survival we have evolved a love of calorie-laden foods that contain fat and sugar. Equally, you will find that children love baked potatoes with butter on top and perhaps a few beans or some cheese. The potato is a fraction of the price of the frozen chip and it retains all the vitamin C content that would be soaked out of it in the process of becoming a chip. The potato contains fewer calories per bite, more fibre, more vitamins and takes minimum preparation time. How? Just put a clean potato in the oven, skin on, for forty minutes and it comes out perfectly baked; crisp on the outside, fluffy on the inside. This, in a nutshell, represents my approach. **Keep things simple but tasty, not processed.**

We can turn our kids' eating habits around. Whether your toddler or your teen is currently overweight, or just tending towards overweight, now is the time to address it. **Teach your kids the language of food.** You are their primary teacher. I was never taught how to cook meals or how to balance my eating as a child or teenager. I did bake, though. I could whip up ninety-six queen cakes (my personal record) by the age of eight and was a dab hand at making all things of a cake and doughnut nature by the age of twelve. However, at eighteen I left home for university unable to make a single nutritious dinner or lunch. I knew nothing of food shopping and budgeting and never bought fruit or vegetables. Why would I, when I could get away with spending my money on biscuits? Balance was not a notion that applied to me.

After a year at college, studying microbiology, eating nothing but pizza and spaghetti Bolognese for dinner and sugar-coated cornflakes for breakfast, I soon realised where poor nutrition was going to lead me. It was only after my summer job waitressing in America that I understood how bleak the future looked for those of us ignorant of good nutrition. I came slowly to the realisation that the reason some families had to wait longer than others to be seated in the breakfast restaurant where I worked was that they were too big to sit at solid booths and could, in fact, only be seated at centre floor tables, where the chairs could be moved to accommodate the extraordinary girth of both parents and children. What compounded my intrigue was that those same families were often the ones who ordered the stack of butter- and maple syrup-drenched pancakes and side of bacon with a 'diet' iced tea.

This was when my passion for nutrition knowledge was ignited. I needed to understand the many myths that confuse our thinking about 'healthy' eating. I decided then and there that my master's degree would be in nutrition. I completed it in 1995, and since graduation I have worked exclusively in the area of nutrition. Today I run two successful weight-loss clinics and deliver corporate in-house nutrition training seminars as well as nutrition lectures to personal trainer students. During my time spent in health promotion with the health board and my previous years in the food supplement industry I became very accustomed to the issues that prevent many of us from achieving balanced daily nutrition. I wrote this book in an attempt to end the confusion for us as parents (I have four kids under the age of ten). **I hope you will find a helpful array of solutions to those problems presented to us by our kids** that will help inform your decisions about food for your family.

This book will not give you quick-fix solutions to your children's actual or potential weight problems. It is not some high-protein spin on nutritional facts, nor does it eliminate sweets, dairy, bread or whatever other food you may yourself have considered cutting out to keep your own weight under control. This book gives you the tools I have found very useful in getting children to eat balanced meals that are calorie-appropriate to their needs, which in itself constantly changes. If you follow the advice in this book **your kids will not be on a diet. They will, instead, get to enjoy good food in a structured and straightforward way.** No gimmicks. No guesswork either.

The following pages will also emphasise something that is all too often overlooked: the importance of regular exercise for the family. Many of us have become very sedentary in recent years. We were not born to be this way: it is only recently that being inactive has become the norm. Our children, too, are often inactive and prone to staying indoors interacting with some electronic gadgetry instead of being outside playing games with other kids. The future for inactive kids is an inactive adulthood, and this equates to a life of battling with overweight. We need to move more, and we need to teach our children how to move. A well-fed, active child will not be an overweight one for long. That child will become fit and healthy, and of an appropriate weight for their height.

We want our children to be healthy. We do our best for their development when it comes to dropping them off and collecting them from activities. We organise their play dates and their social life (which is often better than ours!). We are happy to help with homework. We are willing to spend money on their appearance. Part of this plan must surely involve their being a healthy weight. Overweight kids are more likely to be overweight adults. We do not want this for their future. **While you are still in charge, take this golden opportunity to teach your kids the language of good nutrition and of regular physical exercise so that we can get them back to the way they should be.**

KK424649

Rule 1:

I can say 'No' to food

Our kids are getting fat. We know this. We can see this. They are not getting smaller. They are getting fatter. Worldwide, 42 million children under the age of five are overweight, according to World Health Organisation (WHO) 2010 figures. I can continue to bombard you with figures like these, or you can look around and see for yourself. Our kids are fat. Not all children are overweight, but plenty are. The problem with our complacency on this matter is that we are letting it become normal, by which I mean we are getting accustomed to it. It is quite normal to see overweight kids pottering around today, but we dare not mention it to one another. How many friends would you have left if you mentioned that their kids are fat? We do not want to insult or hurt anyone. Perhaps they are meant to be large, perhaps they are big-boned.

We can console ourselves by looking around to see all the other children of an appropriate weight. And there are plenty of children of a healthy weight pottering around too. I would argue, however, on behalf of those overweight kids who do not want to be heavy, that not even one of them will be happy to be heavier than they should be. They need a voice. Our kids do not want to stand out from the crowd for any reason, least of all for being overweight. Nor do they want to hang out only with other fat kids so as to blend in with their crowd. No, our kids want to be a healthy weight. This should be the norm. It used to be – and not so long ago it was. It needs to be the norm again. Being complacent about our overweight kids is doing them a serious disservice.

If you are reading this book, you are aware of the facts. Whether or not your kids are overweight, reading this book is the first step towards preventing them becoming so in the future. This book is about solutions, not about the many problems facing our overweight children or how bleak their future might look. By the time you come to the end of this book you will not be saddened by the scary facts that abound about our children's future health; you will instead have developed an array of tools and techniques to prevent an overweight future for your children. You will feel confidence in your ability to get your kids back on track to a fantastic future filled with potential. You will also have the knowledge and understanding to help you to continue on the path towards good nutrition and health for yourself. Your entire family, in fact, will benefit over the coming weeks and kick-start their healthiest years ever. If this sounds good to you, turn to the 'instant benefits' in the last chapter now and have a look at what it is you will be working towards.

I put pen to paper on this subject when 'obesity experts' started talking about regularly weighing our children to assess their fat status. This is all wrong, in my opinion. **Kids should never stand on weighing scales. Ever!** Children should remain blissfully unaware of any weight issues that might exist. Children are very smart. They know if you, the parent, have problems maintaining a healthy weight, if you weigh yourself every morning and if you obsess about every morsel of 'bad food' that passes your lips. They know if you are constantly on some sort of 'diet' and

KILKENNY COUNTY LIBRARY

are afraid of eating too much fat or, indeed, any fat. Kids also know themselves if they are overweight, without ever having it spelled out for them: they will feel it. Measuring the facts or getting obsessive about the numbers does not change the facts. On the contrary, it highlights them and brings a child's attention to them at a time when the child does not yet have the skill set to be able to deal with them. That job is ours.

You know the phrase, 'a kid in a sweet shop'? The message of this is that kids cannot control their intake of the nice stuff – sweets – when faced with an endless supply. We are the ones who need to control their intake of 'sweets', whether they are obvious sweet 'treats' or subtle 'breakfast bars' and the like (more on this later). **Our role as parents is to protect our children from harm. Being overweight puts our kids at risk.** Eating too much sugar and fat puts our kids in harm's way. We need to protect them from themselves. We need to protect them from their 'sweet shop' environment. This is our job. They cannot do it for themselves.

I have worked for years with clients on a one-to-one basis for weight loss. Having spent sixteen years discussing food and weight issues with a variety of different people, of all ages and all backgrounds, from New Zealand to Ireland, I can firmly state that highlighting your child's weight 'problem' from an early age will do nothing but set them up to expect to be fat for life. They will always battle with their weight. They will always be on some form of 'diet'. They will always feel fat. How often have I been told, 'I was fat as a child'? More often than I can count. It sets us up as adults to expect only to be fat, for life. It is the excuse we lean on. Our expectations then are, at best, to reduce our weight, but not to be slim, fit, energetic and a healthy weight. No, that is for other people. That is for those who were never fat as children. You may think I exaggerate. I do not. Our expectations arise from our childhood.

When I ask clients what weight they would like to be, they as often as not tell me that of course they would like to be, say, eight stone. When I ask when they last weighed eight stone I am told that they have not seen eight stone register on the scales since they were eleven years old. Then they might say something like, 'Of course I know I will never see eight stone again, I would be happy to get under eleven stone at this age' (and the age in question might be as low as thirty). This might be from a woman who could comfortably achieve eight and a half stone (in this hypothetical case) and have the fitness and excess of available energy to bound out of bed every morning to take on the world. Somehow, however, she will instead settle for a life of being slightly overweight, because she was overweight as a child. We will not dare to expect fitness and the accompanying 'lightness' to be part of our lives if it is an unfamiliar concept to us. We never felt it while we were young, so why should we start looking for it now?

A handful of people will break through this barrier and get to the other side, where they are fit and energised and feeling so good that they would never let go of that feeling again, but this is rare, in my experience. People are, in the main, happy to settle for a weight they feel comfortable with that is just within the healthy range for height – unless, that is, they had a fit younger life. A past sporty type will very often find again their drive and motivation to get fast and fit and feeling fabulous. For many others the concept is an alien one, one they cannot be talked into, as they really do not 'get it'. They never experienced it as kids, so they do not understand how good the pursuit of fitness and a healthy weight can be. This all stems from their youth. Their expectations will have been set when they were younger.

This is a very valuable lesson to spot here and now. Expect your children to be a healthy weight. Follow my guidelines. Apply the learning. If you take this matter in hand, from and including today, your children can be a healthy weight and they may never have to battle with their weight. Of the many tools with which you wish to equip your kids for life, let this be a vital one. Empower first yourself, then your kids, to have full control over weight and fitness. Yes, we all have a certain build – some slight, some heavy – but we can all achieve a lean cover on whatever frame we were given. When our children experience this leanness and fitness they will remember it in later life.

All the lovely clothes in the world, all the toys and holidays, cannot make a child feel as well as the sense of being fit and healthy, light and lithe, energetic and full of beans. For a brief while, you are in charge. At the moment you are the boss. You make the decisions. Your child does what they are told when it comes to wearing their school uniform, or doing their homework, or what time they go to bed. They also need to do what they are told when it comes to food, to achieve balance and to find order where chaos may currently reign. No child will 'get it' straight away. When we learn a new language we have to practise. You would not expect to do a two-day language course and head off to that country fluent in all the nuances of its language. You would expect to practise it repeatedly at home, put it to the test in the country where it is spoken, make many mistakes and correct them as you go along. Getting it very wrong very often is part of the learning process and, as we all know, it is practice that makes perfect.

I am told time and again about kids who simply will not eat what is put in front of them. They are allowed to be finicky about food. They are simply taught bad habits – by us. We give up practising the language of food with them and they stop trying because neither one of us likes to feel that we have failed. They are allowed to have a limited intake of only their favourite foods because we stop repeating the lessons that they need to learn. Repeat the lessons that you will learn in this book on a daily basis. This is how kids learn the language of food.

Remember this as you go. As I say to one of my kids who gets upset at the idea of failing, 'If we stopped trying just because we failed at something, I would have to spend my life carrying you everywhere.' He loves this notion. I tell him the story of a baby who decides, when he tries to walk for the first time in his life, that he has failed because he has fallen down. So his mother has to carry him everywhere for the rest of his life because he has decided he cannot walk, that he has failed. The idea of a 'big boy' being carried around by his ageing mother gets him to see the lighter side every time.

Children learn the language of 'skinny' and 'fat' from the moment they go to school. I wish this were not the case. These are words never used in my house, but they turn up in conversations among my children's friends. They know these words mean something relating to self-esteem. They may not have a full understanding of them, but they have their own interpretation of their importance, in terms of social acceptance. They do not need to have their own possible weight issue pointed out to them: they are not stupid! In my house we talk about being strong, of being powerful, of having strong bones. I find this works to keep the focus on positive pursuits: to be strong enough to climb to the highest point in a tree; to do well at gymnastics; to be the person who never gets caught when playing chase. We never talk of weight loss, of not being allowed to eat sweets, of having to exercise. The terminology used around weight loss is all very negative: the language of loss, misery, hardship. Focus on fun instead. Kids need fun, joy, a light-hearted approach to food. They are, after all, kids.

So put away the weighing scales. Instead, we need to look for ourselves at our own family. Are our children overweight? Yes, if they cannot fit into the age-appropriate clothes in shops; not because they are tall, but because of their waist size. Clothes certainly differ in size from brand to brand; but if no clothes for their age ever fit, look at their waistband. Is it always a problem finding clothes that fit all over? Is their waist too big for the next two sizes up? My GP put it very simply when I complimented him on a photograph above his desk. The photo is of the local swimming pool, taken in the 1960s. I commented on how all the kids looked emaciated by today's standards. In fact, they all looked of a very appropriate weight for height; lean, fit and able-looking. He said that only in the recent ten to fifteen years has he noticed how children have a 'fat pad', as he calls it, around their middle that was never there before, except in a very few children. It seems quite normal now to come across overweight children in his practice.

This is new. The mid-section 'fat pad' that more and more of our children suffer from is a recent development. It is not expected. It does not help them in any way. In fact, it slows them down. It is dangerous to their health. They are carrying around this baggage like a load that weighs them down: it prevents them from running as fast as they might wish to; prevents them from keeping up with their friends; from climbing trees; from generally enjoying their childhood to its fullest. It also puts them at risk of such conditions as type 2 diabetes. Type 2 diabetes, also called 'adult-onset' diabetes, may have to be renamed because so many children globally are now developing it. I do not need to highlight the risks of being an overweight adult: but these risks are significantly higher than average when you are an overweight child. If you are fat as a child you run a great risk of being fat as an adult. Your habits will support a fat lifestyle.

So what do I want to do in this book? I want to give you as many solutions to the problem of overweight children as I can fit into the following pages. You can change this trend right now. It is quite easy, in fact. You will be pleasantly surprised at how easy it will be to apply my recommendations and at how effective they are.

One thing you need to know is that your child might not necessarily need to lose weight. Often, your child will simply grow into the weight he or she already is. This is good news. It means that they will eventually be the appropriate weight for their height and age. Once you make the adjustments to their diet and lifestyle outlined in the following chapters, this will prove very easy indeed. And not a weighing scales in sight! Do not buy a weighing scales if you don't have one. If you do have one, I would respectfully ask you to dig a hole in the garden and bury the thing! Put a little memorial on top to your past relationship with it and to diets and diet products in general, which do not work, which never did work, and which never will work!

I jest.

I do think you should certainly get the thing out of circulation, though. Seriously! Put it under a bed or in the attic. Stop weighing yourself. Never weigh your kids. I meet endless numbers of clients who weigh themselves every day of the week, every week of the year, often many times a day. This can result in a very unhealthy preoccupation with a fluctuation in water weight, which you can do nothing about. Going downstairs to the toaster every morning and asking it, 'How will I feel about myself today?' will provide as relevant an answer as the weighing scales! We are made up of two-thirds water in the first place, and we can fluctuate by up to five pounds a day in water weight. For example, if you consumed a salty meal last night (a Chinese takeaway comes to mind) you might notice that you are heavier on the weighing scales today, by virtue of the amount of water you are retaining. If you have had a bowel movement you are lighter. This is too much information. How do we know when we are losing fat? When our waistband gets looser. What we notice then is a more accurate indication of fat loss, not the instant gratification of water loss, which will go back on when we next eat. The weighing scales can mislead us. Weighing ourselves can become a compulsion that gets us stuck in a rut of fluctuating weight. Clients often describe weight changes to me: they are under the impression that their weight is always in flux, when in fact they just need to step away from the scales and do something else in the morning.

When fat, not water, is lost from the body, however, we notice that we lose a significant amount of fat from our mid-section. This is why obesity experts highlight the importance of waist circum-ference measurements as an accurate indicator of weight gain or loss. For our children the waistband measurement also works very accurately. How do we know when their weight, and therefore health, is improving? When the waistbands on their clothes become looser. If your child loses some excess fat from stores you will see it in the waistband of their trousers or skirt (not necessarily leggings). In my opinion, buttons and zips on clothes are very useful measurement tools, as results shown by structured clothes are not open to interpretation. Our penchant for leisure wear with comfortable waistbands that stretch along with our growing girth is one fashion I am not particularly fond of. We need to do our best to avoid wearing it. Quaint as I sound in saying this, I really think we should get our kids out of leisure gear, at least some of the time, and back into at least the odd 'Sunday best' outfit. This can then be used, perhaps weekly, as the accurate measure you are looking for. My plan might sound a little devious, but I promise I do not intend any deception. I am a scientist and, as such, I like numbers. Numbers are definite. If you can see that your child's waistband has one inch more room in it this week than last, then you have had a successful week. You are getting your child's weight back on the right track.

This is not about fashion. This is about measuring fat. The beauty of fat is that it is all volume. You know the goose fat you can buy at Christmas time for roasting potatoes? If you pick it up from the shelf, it weighs very little. But pick up a fillet steak (which is muscle) and it weighs a lot by comparison. It is dense and heavy, whereas the fat is voluminous and light. And that is why we can always measure fat loss using our clothes. It is easy, it is subtle, your kids won't notice you measuring their success and it is accurate. It is fat we want to lose and only fat – not muscle, not water – so gauge your child's waist circumference in their clothes and you will see whether they are losing weight, gaining, or just holding their own. **Do not use a tape measure.**

One size does not fit all when it comes to clothes, however, as I am well aware. My eight-year-old boy takes age ten in most clothes. He is very tall and broad, but unfortunately for him all the trousers fall down at the waist because he does not have the girth of a ten-year-old. That means he is tall for his age, not overweight. Of course it also means that he has to wear a belt, which he complains about!

So how do we get our kids on the right track again, the track to a healthy weight and a fit body, ready and able to take on the world? By understanding that you are in charge, you are the boss. You pay the bills, you buy the food, and you make the decisions. They do what they are told. Most important, and if you have kids you will know this already: children follow your lead. You lead by example. They do not necessarily do what they are told all the time. They do what they see, for the most part. Kids are great mimics. So if you do not eat dinner at the table, they cannot be expected to always be seated at the table for dinner.

You will often notice in television advertisements for children's food, such as fish fingers, that mothers feed their kids at the table while they themselves potter around, not eating, but watching their kids eat with an air of satisfaction. To me this looks as though they are watching caged monkeys in the zoo at feeding time. I find this odd. It appears to me that feeding our kids has become more of a job to be done than an enjoyable family time. I will be the first to admit that it has taken time, patience and a certain amount of discipline on my part, as much as the children's, to achieve an enjoyable sit-down meal every evening. If you succumb to the notion of feeding the kids on their own, like monkeys, and eating your dinner on your lap while watching television, how long do you think it will be before they expect to be allowed to do the same? My guess is not long at all.

There needs, from today, to be a zero tolerance attitude to this casual approach to eating. It starts with you. In the following chapters you will see that the lessons you teach your kids will be most effectively taught by following them yourself first. They will follow your lead. It is not as tortuous as you might think, and the rewards are many. The good news is that it gets easier and easier and, difficult as it may be to believe now, mealtimes will become pleasant and enjoyable. You will get to the point where you would miss family dinner if you were not there; and you will certainly miss it when the kids get too old to be around for dinner.

Every now and then a prospective client will make an appointment to see me about their overweight child. I always refuse to see the child, but I am happy to consult with the person who makes the call, usually the mother. Why? Because the child is eating what their mother allows them to eat. Many parents, with the best of intentions, try to restrict their child's intake of 'sweets'. It rarely works. Kids can sniff out chocolate, sweets, treats. It is their job! If you think you can restrict a child in a house where there are cupboards full of variety packs, multi-packs, cereal bars and the like, you are wrong. Kids find them. Kids eat them. So I start with the parent. By addressing how the entire household eats, the child's dietary intake changes along with everyone else's. The benefits are endless. Everybody gets to eat good food. Treats are eaten according to agreed schedules. No one eats foods they don't like. Balance becomes the focus and everybody is in it together. One further benefit worth mentioning at this stage is that my approach also involves saving lots of money on the weekly shop. I do not advocate buying special foods, just the kinds of foods you already like to eat.

This is a win-win situation.

It is not a child's fault if they eat too many sweets. I'm sorry to tell you that the fault is ours. We need to change our habits, from buying to 'hiding' sweets and treats, and our children's habits will follow. One of the most important words in our vocabulary when it comes to 'sweets' is 'No'. Your two-year-old learned the power of the word 'No' recently, and they know very well how to use it. We need to use it more too. The answer to the question 'Can I have some?' should be a resounding 'No', unless your plan at that particular time already included some 'treats', for want of a better word. You organise the schedule for the day when it comes to getting to and from school, activities, play dates and television; you also need to be the one to design and adhere to the eating schedule.

> Your two-year-old learned the power of the word 'No' recently, and they know very well how to use it. We need to use it more too. The answer to the question 'Can I have some?' should be a resounding 'No'.

Rule number one, from today, is **I CAN SAY NO TO FOOD** and not be a bad parent. There have to be rules of behaviour about food, the right thing to do and the wrong thing to do. If your five-year-old child asked to stay up late and watch the movie *Jaws*, you would say 'No', and rightly. It is like any other discipline. Saying 'No' to untimely requests for food is the right thing to do. So when your child next asks for the packet of sweets they have just seen at the supermarket checkout, the answer should be 'No'. Do not buy them, do not allow them to be damaged so that they 'have' to be bought; do not entertain the notion of it. You are the boss. The answer is 'No'.

Rule 2:

Eat only at the table

Kids love order and routine. *They* may not know this, but *you* do. They thrive on routine; they understand it and behave best when there is a solid routine in place. Conversely, their behaviour tends to become unpredictable if their routine becomes disturbed. You will know this from experience. You might have memories of trying to get everyone up and out early to go somewhere two weeks into the Christmas holidays, for example. It can be really difficult: one or two can't find their coats or haven't even eaten their breakfast, while another is still in the bathroom playing with toothpaste, having gone in to brush their teeth half an hour ago! Compare this to getting up and off to school every morning during the school term, which is relatively easy because of the routine we have in place.

We are all just big kids. We too thrive on routine. When I first meet clients for weight loss I often spend the first while sorting out their eating schedule. Their eating might be quite ordered during the routine of the working day, for instance, but chaotic at night. The week may be good but it is the weekend that goes pear-shaped. Few people I meet have an orderly relationship with food at all times. And so it is for our children. They might have order at certain times during the day, such as having breakfast at the table at a particular time, lunch and snack time at school and an after-school snack, for instance, but unless a specific schedule is in place for the evening's eating they can end up 'grazing' on bits and pieces for the night. This happens pervasively, over time. It evolves until it becomes a habit and before you know it there is constantly someone buttering toast, scavenging in the fridge or asking for something to eat. Because we may have this habit ourselves we can find it very hard to spot it as a difficulty that needs to be addressed and stopped completely. Our kids would be considerably happier not eating at all for a few hours, busying themselves with other activities until dinner (or supper) time and then sitting down to a good meal with a great appetite for it. If you are the cook in the house you will also feel more successful when plates are cleaned most evenings. There are few things more demotivating when it comes to cooking than having spent time peeling, chopping and preparing, only to notice how little the kids have eaten of your efforts, and how much has gone in the bin.

We all need a schedule around food. We thrive on order. When there are rules around food, order reigns. Order makes life easier and more predictable. An example I might use is my ten-year-old girl's long-fought battle over school lunch. She initially went to school with her perfectly apportioned lunch (or so I thought), but she complained endlessly that all the other girls got sweets and chocolate and biscuits every day; everyone, it seemed, but her. I thought that a treat on Fridays would be an appropriate solution to the problem, but I was wrong. I heard for three long years about packets of biscuits, sausage rolls, jellies, cereal bars and endless other quick-fix calorie bursts being eaten by everyone but her. I stood firm and she got the treat of her choice every Friday, but on Fridays only.

It was difficult, but she understood the rules, so it worked out. In our house you also get treats on Sunday and dessert every night, so rest assured the poor child was not starving.

When my next child (a boy) started school three years later, across the road from the girls' school, there emerged no such issue around treats. Why? The school has a written lunch box policy that you agree to before your child starts there. The policy states that 'treats' are to be brought to school on Fridays only. As a result, my son has never once asked for a treat on other days of the week. In fact, if a home-made wholemeal banana muffin turns up in his lunch box, on occasion, he will often return it uneaten, for fear of it being a treat. He loves the rules. He understands the rules. The authorities have set down these rules, so he does not question them. The norm in his school supports this message and it is reinforced at home by me. In fact, it makes it a lot easier on his older sister, too, knowing that her strict mum did not just invent the 'Friday only' rule on a whim. Now none of the kids questions this rule any more; they just follow it.

So kids love rules. We are the authorities. You, as a parent, are top dog. You make the rules. We need to have rules around food, as we do around other behaviours. I'm sure you have rules about spitting or fighting or putting away toys or tidying bedrooms. So, too, you should impose rules about food. This is not a dictatorship I am talking about. Kids need choice in what they eat, of course; but there should, from today, be order around food with eating schedules that are adhered to.

My rule number two is: **EAT ONLY AT THE TABLE**. In other words, 'If your bum's not on a seat, you don't eat!' If this were the only rule you adhered to, it could significantly change your child's habits around food, and for life. When I meet clients, I find that this is one of the biggest contributors to their problems of overweight. Our habits have become very sloppy around food. We often just make it up as we go along. We can cook a few different meals a day, depending on who's eating what and when and quite often we will eat in front of the television, or at a counter-top, because it is convenient. We may not have any table manners or rules that need to be adhered to. We tend often to simply go with the flow of whatever is happening that evening. Other events might take priority over mealtime, from television programmes to dropping and collecting kids, or there might be sheer lack of interest, mixed with a little laziness on our part.

It might come across as antiquated, but I strongly believe that we need to resurrect some old-fashioned values when it comes to food. We need set mealtimes and, ideally, we need to eat together as a family.

Regardless of whether this is always achievable, there should be the golden rule of 'eat only at the table' for your children, every time, with no exceptions. They can sit even if you are not sitting with them. I do suggest at least having a cup of tea at the table with them while they eat their supper, if yours is later.

I might go back to the idea of feeding time at the zoo as an approach to feeding our kids, which I think should stay in the zoo! Our kids need the respect shown to them in your taking time to actually sit with them, even if it is just to broker peace, and, in time, ideally, to have a conversation. At the very least, lead by example, in showing them how it is done. If you sit, they will happily sit with you, and they won't get up every two minutes to walk around to pick up toys between bites of food. You might find this an impossible task in the morning when you are rushing and racing to get everyone out to school and to work; you may relish your lunch in splendid isolation and silence before collecting the horde from school. Make no apologies for this: you deserve a break from the noise, on occasion. What I am talking about, primarily, is what might be described as the main meal of the day. For most of us that is dinner in the evening; it may very well be lunchtime in your house. The details do not matter: it is the principle I want to get across here; that we sit down together, perhaps just once in the day, and eat.

There should be a certain formality attached to these proceedings. Toys, phones and any kind of electronic device should be banned from the table at mealtime. The table should be set. There should be no playing with food allowed; just eating and conversation. And if a child wants to play or watch television, they should eat up and leave the table to do just that, if it has been agreed to.

Involve your children in setting up for mealtime. Mine love it. One will set the table (depending on who gets picked) and, as a reward, he or she is the one who decides that day where everything goes and where everyone sits. Simplistic as this might sound, it is the feeling of empowerment that attracts my kids to this task. If you set the table for dinner you get to choose where everybody sits that day. Could this approach be too simple to be successful? Try it. Then you will see its simple charm.

Having the correct cutlery also helps – smaller spoons for smaller people, and each child's preferred cup – but kids also love to emulate their parents' habits, so the bigger ones will really want the same knife and fork you use yourself. Again, this might sound stupidly simple, but when you challenge, say, an eight-year-old to use a knife and fork correctly (knife in the right hand, not fork; leave that to American films!) he or she will take on the challenge and enjoy the juggling and fun of chasing a pea around the plate with a knife and fork. Like eating rice with chopsticks for us, as adults – if we are not used to using them – for a child, a knife and fork can present endless opportunities to make the mess they wanted to in the first place. Notice, though, that they will eat their vegetables, albeit messily, and enjoy the process, not gulp down only a handful of chips for tea.

Formal as my next proposal will seem to you, stay with me for a minute! I aim (not always successfully) to put a tablecloth on the table for Sunday dinner most weeks. Daft, you may think. Do you really want the extra laundry on a Monday morning? I think my answer to that question is yes. Why not? Life is short. Why not make just one meal a week really special? Besides, my tablecloth of choice is the fastest-drying thing in my laundry basket and takes a total of two minutes' effort on my part to process (and in reality it only gets washed every second week). You might wonder why I bother to do this. The reason is that I simply love Christmas and everything to do with it. When we lived in New Zealand for three winters, my husband and I greatly missed Christmas. Yes, Christmas goes ahead every year, but in Auckland Christmas took place in high summer, at a daily temperature of about 28°C. We took our summer holidays at Christmas. On St Stephen's Day we went north to the Bay of Islands in our shorts to eat barbecued turkey, ham and plum pudding leftovers.

All winter long, however (April until November, it seemed), we had none of the lift or distraction of the lead-up to and eventual celebration of Christmas. I really missed that.

Back in Ireland I begin Christmas preparations in November, between making two cakes and five plum puddings, and putting up lights and decorations (far too early, according to some family members, who shall remain nameless). This distraction reminds me so much of my youth. Over the much shorter version of Christmas we did in the 1980s, what I remember most is setting the Christmas table. I was the one who washed the good delph in time for Christmas, just after the school holidays started. I was also the one who laid the tablecloths on the table and dusted down the dining room for its annual exposure to family life. What we did after Christmas Day was to leave the table fully set for the week until and including New Year's Day dinner. I loved that. The formality of the special ware, used even for breakfast, in this formal setting, meant celebration, holidays and some special feelings. Now I do an extreme version of this. Thus, in my house, the table stays set until and including 6 January (the tablecloths being washed once or twice for the duration); and I extend this for a lot of the year into Sunday dinner time too. Why not? What I hope to promote, in doing this, is a joy of eating at the table with family. We do not walk around the house eating.

We sit. Trust me, it does not always work out so beautifully: on occasion someone will pout, argue or not like their dinner, and that's just the adults! For the most part, however, it genuinely works and it is joyous and fun.

My father, at eighty-eight years of age, would find it impossible to walk down the street eating an apple. He couldn't do it. He will eat an apple on a plate, carefully cut into quarters, at a scheduled snack time. Seriously. The formality that exists for him about food means that I know I can phone him and find him just about to sit down to lunch at one p.m. exactly, just as the lunchtime radio news begins. I do not exaggerate. Tea is at six-thirty: never earlier; never later. I could offer the man a cup of tea and a slice of cake at five o'clock and he would not accept, since he would shortly be going home for his tea. While it is regimented, this eating schedule means that he eats an appropriate amount every day and never becomes overweight. He learned this habit in childhood and it stuck. No hunger, just habit. He will claim to have been underfed and hungry at boarding school. This was very likely to have been the case and it would have taught him to value each meal rather than squander it as our kids might today. To watch the man slice his bread into bite-sized morsels before buttering and eating it, as a result of such a disciplined approach, is nothing short of inspiring, though. He can, if you believe it possible, leave perhaps an eighth of a slice of bread on his plate uneaten and put it into the breadbin for tomorrow, if his appetite has been satisfied on less than that full slice of bread. This training came early in his life, from a strict, frugal upbringing and enforced table manners at the school dinner table.

I am not suggesting we cut our bread into matchbox-sized pieces to eat, not for our kids. Life is short enough! I do, however, feel that we should be tuned into our appetite enough to feel able to leave a few bites behind, and we need to pass this skill on to our kids. No school will do that job for us today. When you address your food with such formality and you respect mealtimes to this extent you would be amazed at how conscious you become of the amount of food you are eating. It makes it much easier, too, for your kids to control the amount of food they consume in one sitting when there is a degree of formality around eating. When they are not distracted by toys, arguments with their siblings or, indeed, the television, they can focus on their feelings of hunger and satiety (fullness). Whenever one of the kids at my table is acting up they do time on the stairs, I'm afraid. Disputes are not allowed to happen at the table. After years of enforcing this rule I would have to say that rows rarely, if ever, happen in our house at mealtime any more. Arguments happen aplenty, just not at the dinner table.

My father, at eighty-eight years of age, would
find it impossible to walk down the street
eating an apple. He couldn't do it. He will eat
an apple on a plate, carefully cut into quarters,
at a scheduled snack time.

I also think that we should never allow ourselves or
our kids to eat 'on the hoof'. How often do you find
yourself eating bits and pieces at the counter-top while
making sandwiches for lunchboxes? I can easily get
into the habit of following the 'one for me, one for you,
one for me' rule that has me picking bits off the corner
of each slice of bread. I love the blackened crust on
hand-made white loaves, while the kids dislike the
black bits, so this is a win-win situation, as long as
there is plenty of butter around. Unless I enforce the 'if
my bum's not on a seat I don't eat' rule, this could go
on all evening, on a particular day, especially if a few
hormones are thrown into the mix. The same applies
to our kids. If they are allowed to graze all day, picking
up a cheese slice one minute, a biscuit the next, or a
glass of orange juice the next, they will never listen
closely enough to their appetite to learn how *not* to
overeat. Think about it: if you never feel hunger, which
I describe as a rumble in your tummy, you will never
spot the feeling of being full and nicely satisfied.

The Japanese describe this feeling as the principle of leaving the table at eighty per cent full. This works because you allow yourself at least twenty minutes, ideally forty, to feel completely full. If you leave the table at a hundred per cent full, twenty minutes later you will be fit for very little other than a nap. It takes at least twenty minutes for our brain to get those 'full' signals from our stomach nerves. This is a great trick or tool to use. When used in reverse, I find it fabulously accurate in gauging a child's hunger level. I will often ask my kids before dinner time, 'How hungry are you, on a scale of one to ten?' If the answer is four (say because they had a late snack due to activities or a birthday party) I might put dinner off for half an hour. If the answer is nine, I know that they will eat plenty of vegetables that day, so I might put extra on their plates. The idea here is that we should aim never to stray above eight or nine, when they are starving and prone to eating anything to quell their hunger; or to be over eighty per cent full.

In other words, if our kids are allowed to eat when they are not truly hungry, because they happen to have opened the fridge and something caught their eye, they are, by definition, overeating. When they next sit down to a meal they are almost certainly going to eat more calories than are needed that day. These represent calories that, if they are not used up, must eventually be stored in fat cells. If your kids do this regularly, they will become overweight. It is that easy, I'm afraid. If any one of us, adult or child, consumes a paltry 100kcal (kilocalories) more than are used in a day, in thirty-five days we will have gained one pound of fat. Why? There are 3,500kcal in a pound of fat. This is a scary scientific fact. So if your child has put on a pound of fat in approximately one month they might simply have eaten one too many slices of bread, very lightly buttered (coming in at about 100kcal) on a regular basis. Imagine the damage, from a calorie perspective, that could be done if that child were allowed free reign over the 'goodies' cupboard. Remember, kids smell treats, kids find treats, kids eat treats. So if your household contains a stash of treats, from potato chips to chocolate to biscuit bars, your kids will know where they are hidden and they will eat them, on the hoof, between meals and at every opportunity. This ends up clouding their judgement when it comes to feelings of hunger and satisfaction. When this habit takes hold, weight gain follows. When a formal meal schedule is set and they are allowed such treats only at the end of a meal or only on Fridays, or whatever system might suit your family, as long as it is predictable and scheduled, the kids will not need to go in search of 'forbidden' treats. When treats are allowed, but scheduled, no such need exists. Our kids are more likely to resist over-eating them and you can control their intake by giving an appropriate portion of treat foods at the end of mealtime, as dessert (more on this subject later).

What you would also observe if you were to watch how my father eats, as an example personified of formality around food, is that on some days he eats a big tea and on others a very small one. Just because the timing is set does not mean he eats a set amount every day. He will eat according to his level of hunger. This will relate to his activity levels on that particular day or week, whether he has been cutting the lawn or out dancing or taking a longer walk than usual.

If I were to give an example of what 'not' to do, it would be this: eating at the cinema or while watching television. For example, if you're sitting in front of the cinema screen with a great big 'family-sized' bag of sweets (they are never small at the cinema), your brain won't really register whether you eat one or forty-one sweets. Why? Because you are distracted by what's going on in the movie. Your brain is up there on the screen engaged and enthralled by the plot; your sweets are simply being shovelled into your mouth. You know you will finish them; as soon as you start they are as good as gone! This is what we also tend to do at home. Our kids eat while watching television. Not only do they overeat in these circumstances, but the television is full of food ads, not by coincidence. One ad for a product is directed at them and there is another version directed at you. Between the constant pleas

from your kids and the constantly reinforced messages
directed towards you, these products sell very well.
How often have you bought a yoghurt drink, for
example, on the back of such a campaign? These ads
create the desire to buy and thus eat more food. Part of
the function of advertising is to create the perception
of a need where previously there was none. When
these products are in the house they get eaten. When
they get eaten they are often eaten over and above what
would have previously been a normal day's calorie
intake. Again, I urge you to think about that simple
excess of 100kcal per day making a quick pound of
excess body fat.

Order around food means that mealtimes are set,
snack times are regular and scheduled. When children
know this, you don't have to keep making up new
rules and schedules because of changing circumstances. If your teenager wants to stay in bed until
eleven-thirty on a Saturday, then great: they are
growing, after all, and need to reserve some energy for
that task. However, they have missed breakfast. It is
now a lot closer to lunchtime, which might be at one
o'clock. What they might eat now is a small snack,
such as fruit and yoghurt, that would be similar to
what and when they would have eaten all week at
school, thus not spoiling their appetite for lunch at
one. What you will then find is that they are first at the
table for lunch, hungry, enthusiastic and happy to

consume perhaps soup and a sandwich, which would not have had the same appeal if they had had toast and cereal at noon. If your family always has dinner at six, then when one of the kids comes looking for something at five you are in a position to say 'No, dinner is at six.' 'No' is the word. They will not go hungry. We live in a time of plenty. Our child had lunch a couple of hours ago and is about to eat again in a little while. They will not die of hunger. We need to get back to the basics, which, in this case, means that we need an appetite for dinner; that is when broccoli begins to look good again and all the vegetables get cleaned off the plate, before any talk of dessert.

You already know all this from experience. I am simply reminding you. You know that when your kids have eaten a little while ago, because someone opened the fridge and found a yoghurt drink, they are not interested in eating their vegetables. Instead, they pick at the crust on the fish finger, eat some beans, and leave the greens untouched! You can probably also remember a day, say when it snowed, when you had to drag them in for dinner, wet, hungry and exhausted. They finished their dinner that day, greens and all. Spot the difference. We can recreate those circumstances and that appetite for good food every single day by saying 'No' to snacks that are not scheduled. They will get the hang of the new rules very quickly.

Why? Because kids love order and routine. They thrive on it. You are not a bad parent if you say 'No' to unscheduled snacks, if you resist the wails of 'But I'm hungry!' You are doing brilliantly in getting them to eat an old-fashioned square meal. I will discuss the specific shape of this meal in a later chapter. I can remember very clearly being shooed out of the kitchen as a child if I asked for the merest morsel, even an apple, up to an hour before dinner. We never ate 'on the hoof', we sat. Our kids need to sit down to eat.

Rule 3:

Have they had their fruit and vegetables today?

I have yet to meet a person who eats the recommended amount of fruit and vegetables, every day, when they initially come to see me. Our expectations about how much we should eat are too low. We fail to achieve the WHO's recommendations for the daily intake of fruit and vegetables. We might do poorly some days, well on some other days, but I have never met anyone who does well seven days a week, every week of the year. This, to me, represents one of the primary reasons they have ended up overweight and thus feel the need to consult me in the first place. My first job of work with most of my clients is to get them into the habit of eating far more fruit and vegetables than they are used to.

There is currently a strong trend to move away from eating too many carbohydrates. This means that great immediate weight loss is achieved (not necessarily all fat – much of this is water, as discussed earlier), but there are poor adherence rates to the plan in the longer term. You will see this trend in all the high-protein plans in women's magazines and diet books being sold at the moment. This is simply food fashion. The movement away from carbohydrates means a move away from too much consumption of fruit, along with breads, cakes and pasta. Thus, many people I meet are nervous about eating too much fruit. I like to remind clients that the instigator of such high-protein, low-carbohydrate eating as a means to rapid weight loss, Dr Atkins, suffered many heart attacks in his latter years. My point being that all such quick-fix approaches to fat loss tend to be short-lived in their success and nature has it that after any such 'famine' we will always want to 'feast'. This means that the person who quickly loses ten pounds in one week following this type of diet will put those ten pounds back on in the following week, once normal eating is resumed. This is something I see all the time.

Mainstream science stands firmly behind the notion that carbohydrates are our primary source of fuel: they are the petrol in our engine. Fifty-five to sixty per cent of our daily calories should be in the form of carbohydrates, and we need to eat plenty of those carbs in the form of fruit and vegetables. I take my cue from the WHO when it comes to making recommendations, and they currently recommend that we eat between five and thirteen portions of fruit and vegetables every day of the week, every week of the year. These numbers may seem a little frightening at first. On the contrary, this is good news. **Get the fruit bowl back out of cold storage and fill it up with all your and your kids' favourite fruits.**

I love the Australian way of interpreting these recommendations. They say that 'two plus five' portions of fruit and vegetables, respectively, is the way forward. I like the simplicity of this interpretation for our kids. In fact, the WHO says that a minimum standard of 400g of fruit and vegetables should be eaten by each and every one of us every day of the week. On my weighing scales that equates to, for example, an average-sized kiwi fruit, a small apple, a portion of broccoli, a portion of carrots and a tomato. This, remember, is considered to be our minimum standard, so it is a good goal for achieving with your kids. In practice, we eat nothing like this amount of fruit and vegetables – unless you are reading this book in France, Italy, Austria, Germany or perhaps Poland.

How much is enough? In Ireland, our recommendations stand at 'five plus' fruit and vegetables a day. This is not enough. If we regularly achieved five plus portions of fruit and vegetables a day, I believe we would be doing very well. But I prefer the WHO recommended average of five to thirteen portions per day for the average person. Why? Because it means we pretty much need to start our day with fruit, end our day with fruit and fill all the gaps with fruit, so as to regularly achieve this. The WHO actually suggests that we have either fruit or vegetables with every meal. And these are good habits to form. These recommendations are for adults, but they also apply to children from the age of six upwards.

Does your child achieve five to thirteen portions of fruit and vegetables per day? I doubt it if you are still reading this book! Few do. Children under the age of six need less bulk than this, yet the habit of eating little portions or 'tasters' of fruit and vegetables at snack time is one that can begin as soon as a child begins eating solids. If we start with small amounts, we can work our way up to considerably more by the time the child reaches the age of six. As the WHO puts it, as kids approach school age they should gradually move to a diet that is lower in fat and higher in fibre. Of course, fats should come from nutritious sources, such as oily fish, olive oil, meat and dairy products, not from snack foods such as chocolate, biscuits and crackers, but we will discuss this fully later.

Cucumber slices are one of my six-year-old girl's favourite lunchbox fillers. Recently, we discovered baby bite-sized cucumbers in our local shop and suddenly my four-year-old started to eat them too. Anything 'fun-sized' tends to appeal greatly to kids. I very often do carrot sticks before dinner, as the children are getting hungry and are sitting down waiting for their food. In my house broccoli is called 'starters'. Daft as this may sound, it works. Often, one of my kids will ask, 'What are we having for starters?' It sounds very posh indeed, starters on a Monday evening, but this is a trick I have used for many years now, with great success, to get them to try new vegetables. They might eat their broccoli and carrots, but not all of them will eat sugar-snap peas, or baby corn. When they get just one or two pieces as a 'starter' and they are hungry, you would be surprised at how much they will try. So experiment: introduce a new vegetable every week or so. Providing just a piece or two per child, once a week, means they can take it or leave it, but they will recognise it again the next time it turns up and won't be horrified at the sight of it. Three out of my four kids eat Brussels sprouts now, which I am delighted about, not because the Brussels sprout is any magic elixir for health but because it shows how effective these simple methods are. The only reason child number four has not yet bought into the beauty of these little green beasts is that he is still four and not yet ready to toe the line. My money is on him eating them by the age of five!

It is a little-known fact that kids say 'No' to anything new – that isn't ice cream of course – up to a dozen times before they will say 'Yes'. Mangetout is a recent addition to my four-year-old son's repertoire, for instance, after about a year and a half of refusing to put one near his lips! We should keep introducing little bits of new vegetables and fruit on a regular basis so as to keep children's food horizons broad. Vegetable and dip combinations can also interest some children. Hummus, for instance, in all its garlicky goodness, is loved by two of mine and disliked intensely by the other two – so far. Salsa is another dip that can be used to get your kids to try such things as celery sticks. Keep it fun. Get your child involved. Bring them (occasionally) to the shop with you to help you choose which vegetable they might be willing to try next. Try an either/or approach, I would never recommend asking a young child an open question like, 'Which vegetable will we try today?' I am much more in favour of such questions as, 'Will we try orange tomatoes today or baby corn?'

It is a little-known fact that kids say 'No' to anything new – that isn't ice cream of course – up to a dozen times before they will say 'Yes'. Mangetout is a recent addition to my four-year-old son's repertoire, for instance, after about a year and a half of refusing to put one near his lips!

Soups are another great delivery system for vegetables. I am not a huge fan of supermarket bought soups as they tend to be extremely salty, which can be too much to give a small child on a regular basis (kids' bodies are smaller than ours, so they need less salt). Some years back I bought a hand-held blender, which inspired me to delve into the world of soup-making. Suddenly I was able to whip up (literally) a carrot and coriander soup in ten minutes and a sweet tomato and basil soup in even less time. I tend now, in winter, to make a large vat of soup on a Monday (my day off because I work on Saturdays) to have for the week. I will admit that my kids don't exactly fight over who gets the soup first – they are not huge fans of the stuff – but I find that as an after-school snack, maybe three out of the five days, they are pretty glad to have a warm cup of it placed in their hands before they get down to the grind of homework. Just recently, my middle boy came home a little unwell from school at the end of his day. Tired and a little sad, he reported that he had been sitting by the heater earlier that day in school feeling unwell and he dreamed of coming home to some hot tomato soup and cheese on toast. I thought that was the cutest thing ever. Not only did he want the comfort of home but he also wanted the warmth of a cup of soup, and not any soup, my tomato soup! I was delighted both for him and, of course, for myself and my efforts on the soup front. My trick when making something like soup for kids is to make it sweet. Kids are drawn to all things sweet; they cannot help themselves. The preference for sweet represents the human instinct for survival: searching for something sweet to eat means searching for calories, which can protect you against starvation and, in evolutionary terms, extinction. (So much in such a small bowl of soup!) My carrot and coriander soup is sweet because I use organic carrots (the one time I always buy organic) and my tomato soup is sweet because I add a little sugar to the tomatoes while they are cooking, to take away the acidic edge that kids detest.

Five-minute Carrot and Coriander Soup

This soup takes five minutes of your time to make. That's it. It takes another ten minutes' boiling time.

Ingredients

✓ I tablespoon olive oil

✓ I onion, peeled and chopped

✓ I bag (750g) of organic carrots, peeled and chopped

✓ I stock cube (chicken or vegetable) or 500ml home-made chicken stock, for those dedicated to the cause!

✓ a small bunch of coriander

✓ salt and pepper

Method

• Simply pour the olive oil into a big saucepan and add the chopped onion. Cook over a gentle heat. During this three to five minutes, peel and chop your carrots: this is the only hard labour involved. I have tried using unpeeled carrots in this soup. Believe me, it does not work. It comes out stringy and horrible and no one eats it.

• By the time the carrots are peeled and chopped it is time to add them to the pot, along with the stock cube and 500ml of boiling water or your 500ml of pre-made stock. The choice is yours. (I do make chicken stock on occasion and it is truly lovely in any soup recipe.)

• Allow the soup to bubble away for about ten minutes, then add a little fresh coriander (you can omit the coriander if you forgot to buy it: the result will still be delicious) and go in with your hand-held blender to make a lovely smooth, velvety soup. Of course a stand-alone liquidiser will do the job beautifully too, but with a considerable difference to the washing-up. A hand-held blender really removes that barrier to success.

- I serve this soup with some brown soda bread and cheese for an after-school snack or for a Saturday lunch after football training on a cold day. Wonderful! For the parents this can benefit from a little extra salt and pepper with, perhaps, some extra coriander on top.

෨෬

Smooth Sweet Tomato and Basil Soup

Successful children's soups need to be super-smooth. You will find that they turn their noses up at anything with 'bits' in it. Simple as this principle is, if you adhere to it, you can have great success getting your kids to eat a wide variety of soups and sauces.

Ingredients

✓ I tablespoon olive oil

✓ I onion, peeled and chopped

✓ Ikg tomatoes (any type)

✓ I stock cube (vegetable or chicken)

✓ I heaped teaspoon tomato purée

✓ I teaspoon sugar

✓ salt and pepper

✓ a small bunch of fresh basil

✓ ½ cup milk

Method

• Pour the olive oil into a large saucepan and add the chopped onion. Cook gently for three to five minutes while you coarsely chop the tomatoes. I use any tomatoes I find in my fridge – small, large, ugly or cute. In fact, this soup usually comes about because I am looking at an uneaten load of tomatoes that are past their best, and need to use them up. Those tomatoes make the best soup, in my opinion. As soon as they are chopped, add them to the saucepan and your labour is almost at an end.

- Add the stock cube with 500ml boiling water, the tomato purée, the sugar, a little pepper and a little salt and allow it to simmer for about ten minutes. After this time, add the basil and blitz until smooth. Add the milk to serve.

- Kids love the slight sweetness and slight creaminess of this light, nutritious soup.

ళ఼ఞ

As for fruit, I meet a lot of mothers who claim that their kids 'hate' fruit. I find it hard to imagine that a child could dislike all fruit all the time. There is such a vast array of choice, texture, colour, size and fun to be had with fruit. If your child won't eat an apple, fine. What about grapes? Have you ever frozen a grape? Kids love experimenting with these concepts. Get your child to put a bunch of grapes in the freezer and monitor its progress until the grapes are frozen and crisp. They're very likely to eat them if you describe them as chewy, crunchy sweets crossed with a piece of fruit! A child will find it hard to resist the super sweetness of an over-ripe pineapple. I buy them when they are at their ripest, which is also when they are nearing their best-before date and therefore at their cheapest. Chopped into little pieces and put in a bowl on the table at snack-time, it is gone in a flash. Ripest is nicest in our house! Blueberries are lovely for picking at; kiwis are fantastic fun when eaten out of an eggcup with a spoon; you can sometimes find tiny bananas, the size of your thumb. You will find that children love the novelty of these fun-sized foods. Though they might seem like little morsels to you and you might wonder if it is worth the bother, it is their tolerance of these foods that you are chasing at this stage.

What they tend to get very bored with quickly is the great big apple in the lunchbox or the banana the size of their arm. They may feel daunted by the idea of having to finish it all in one sitting, plus they very often do not get adequate time at lunch break to eat all of it and they want to be in the yard playing instead. This is a very common complaint I hear from parents regarding left-over fruit in lunchboxes. Keep it small, keep it fun. Grapes and a sliced-up kiwi fruit can be eaten a lot faster than one enormous Granny Smith.

Dessert every day is another tool (or trick) I use to get my children to eat more fruit, and it works. Other kids are always amazed that in our house we have a daily dessert, not reserved just for weekends or special occasions. Even their cousins are jealous of the idea. Dessert, however, in our house, comprises something from the milk group (i.e. custard, yoghurt or ice cream) and fruit, and that's it. The kids do not spot my healthy intent, and neither do the visiting kids on play dates, nor the cousins who might stay for a week. None of them knows my methods. All they see is dessert on the counter-top waiting for them after they have eaten their main course. Now, the fruit can be stewed apple one day, tinned fruit cocktail the next, or fresh strawberries or defrosted frozen berries with bite-sized meringues, grapes or sliced pear with chocolate shavings, so the kids cannot spot the trend of the two main ingredients in all desserts all the time.

Kids actually love fruit. They love the idea of dessert every day. Marry the two. Why? Because we are born to love the taste of 'sweet' foods. It is pure instinct. Breast milk is sweet, and our quest for sweetness continues long after the breastfeeding phase. When you choose sweet (that means ripe) fruit and present it to your child in a number of fun ways you will find that they too love fruit. They were born to. Is there a child out there who would not enjoy the mess and taste involved in dipping a strawberry, grape, slice of banana or apple into warm chocolate sauce every once in a while? (A day you do not have the tablecloth on might be the one.) Yes, this is a little perfectionist, I admit. Most of us do not have enough time in the day to slice up an apple, let alone melt chocolate and start messing around with skewers and the like. My point, however, is that there are many ways of getting your child interested again (or for the first time) in eating enough fruit every day, consistently.

So let's look at how you can introduce four fruit hits a day and another four vegetable injections into your child's schedule to get a method of achieving their recommended daily intake.

A fruit snack mid-morning is a key factor. Get them to like fruit by working with their appetite. When a child is hungry, fruit looks good to them; and when they are full, chocolate looks good. A mandarin orange, a plum or a few strawberries: anything bite-sized tends to work, I find. Incidentally, it is important to include this snack on non-school days as well, otherwise the toaster goes on and the drip-feed begins, or they are looking into the fridge with intent.

Mid-afternoon is another important opportunity we should aim never to miss to get fruit past their lips. When they come in from school, it will be snack time, of course, and this snack should always contain some fruit where possible. For instance, banana on toast, apple with yoghurt or fruit salad with orange juice poured over it.

They can get a third fruit hit after dinner in the form of dessert with something milky, as discussed above, and if they are hungry again later you can give them another little fruit shot as part of their bed-time snack. Raisins, chopped apple and chopped pineapple are great night-time favourites in my house. Anything sweet and pre-peeled, in fact, appeals, as the work is taken out of it for them. Put in a bowl and placed in front of them with a fork sticking out of it, they find it difficult to resist. I know it might sound as though you need to spoon-feed your kids, but while I am advocating that, yes, initially you place the stuff into their hands, in no time at all they will come looking for it themselves, when their habits are up and running. It takes three weeks to form a habit, so stick with it for a little while and it will get a lot easier over the weeks.

Stewed Blood Fruit and Custard

This recipe evolved – as the best recipes often do – because I wanted to use up uneaten fruit. It is great fun, looks great and with a name like 'blood fruit', really piques the interest of even the pickiest child.

Ingredients

- ✓ I bag (say 1kg) apples, such as Granny Smith, Bramley, Cox's Pippin
- ✓ ½ packet frozen berries (e.g. blackberries, blueberries, strawberries, red berries or a mixture) or left-over fresh berries
- ✓ custard powder
- ✓ sugar
- ✓ vanilla extract
- ✓ milk

Method

- Pour a little water into the bottom of a large saucepan. While it comes to the boil, peel and chop the apples, then add them to the water. Allow it to come back to the boil and simmer gently for about ten minutes. Then add the frozen berries and stir through. Turn off the heat and allow it to sit while you make the custard.

- Make the custard according to the instructions on the packet, perhaps with a little less sugar than recommended. Add a few drops of vanilla extract, which really adds a delicious flavour.

- Stewed fruit and custard can be served as dessert or for an afternoon snack. I tend to make plenty of stewed fruit at the one time so that I can have some cold fruit 'compote' in the fridge, which goes beautifully on muesli in the mornings with plain or vanilla-flavoured yoghurt. The fruit can be re-heated in the microwave and served with some vanilla ice cream another day. A most lovely combination!

ೲೲ

The vegetable battle strikes fear into most parents, in my experience. I can reassure you that it can be very simply won, with a little perseverance. What we may not understand is that no one vegetable has to be eaten to achieve health for your children. Your child may never eat broccoli. That is fine. Your kids, however, may love ham and cabbage. Anything green will do. Perhaps they like their sugar-snaps raw? Great. Don't get bogged down into thinking that if they won't touch spinach, they will eat nothing green; they may surprise you and take a liking to roasted Brussels sprouts at Christmas. It happens. What *not* to do is get your child in a head-lock and make them eat their vegetables all in the one sitting.

When he was growing up my husband was made to eat turnip, which he detested. He would have been very happy to eat it raw, but was never allowed to. If he swiped a little from the chopping-board he got into serious trouble. His parents meant well, but the result of his being made to eat turnip at dinner time, again and again, and the ensuing bad feeling that would surround the war zone that dinner seemed to him on turnip days means that, to this day, if I cook turnip as part of any dinner he can smell it before he is out of the car in the driveway. He will somehow be drawn to lift the lid off the pot containing the offending root and run a mile from dinner that evening until all the turnip has cooled down on the plates. If he were not interested in the rest of dinner he would keep running!

The lesson to be learned from this extreme vegetable story is to take a 'little and often' approach to a wide variety of vegetables with your kids. Introduce one Brussels sprout on the plate every now and again along with their favourite vegetables, for instance. The supermarkets are great at packaging tiny amounts of vegetable combinations, enough for everyone to try just a few morsels from the one packet. Remember that frozen vegetables are every bit as good as fresh, nutrient-wise, once the fresh have sat around for a few days in the shop and in your kitchen.

We should also, ideally, eat something orange every day. Carrots are easy. I buy mine organic, as they are fantastically sweet in comparison to the non-organic, and there is very little difference in the price. Whether you eat them peeled, raw, cooked, liquidised in curries or as a starter does not matter. I liquidise carrots and put them into children's curry. The resulting sauce is sweet and voluminous and the kids love it. I use the same pot that I first boiled the carrots in to cook the rice, so there's no extra washing-up and my magic hand-held blender takes nothing more than a rinse to clean. Easy!

If not carrots, why not try sweet potato? Roast one with the roast potatoes or try them chipped. I even do potato crisps on occasion, using both ordinary potatoes and sweet potatoes and a tablespoon or two of olive oil. There are no complaints that day.

Perhaps you might put raw yellow pepper into a lunchbox. I do put a vegetable portion into the children's lunchboxes every day, incidentally; otherwise I find they will not achieve their five hits a day. A few baby tomatoes (fruit, officially) with sliced peppers works for one of my kids. Carrot sticks works for another. Another will actually ask for raw broccoli – who saw that coming?

Whether it is vegetable soup, salad or mashed vegetables that your kids eat for lunch and for dinner every day, eating vegetables twice daily will be one of those invaluable habits they learn now and that will continue into the future. Wouldn't you be delighted to think, in the future, that you equipped your twenty-something son or daughter, living in their first apartment and starting their first job, with the skills and interest in vegetables to be able to master a vegetable-filled curry in a flash or, indeed, to make a weekly pot of vegetable soup?

We are creatures of habit. **The great habits around fruit and vegetables that you put an effort into instilling in your child now will stick for life.** This is all good. They eat well now and, best of all, they will, as a result, never have to battle with their weight as an adult. I can guarantee it. Trust me, when I meet overweight adults I find that they do not eat enough fruit and vegetables, they don't even come close to eating enough, not by a long shot.

Kids' Curry

This curry came about as the result of having picky kids over to our house, who appeared to like nothing I cooked. Instead of being mortally insulted by the constant refusal to eat anything vaguely resembling a vegetable that I might put on a dinner plate, I took up the challenge. I can now practically guarantee that even the choosiest child will adore this curry. Do try it. This recipe serves four hungry or six small kids.

Ingredients

✓ 500g (approx.) carrots, peeled and chopped

✓ I onion, peeled and chopped

✓ 3 chicken breasts or 4 chicken thighs, chopped into very small pieces

✓ 2 tablespoons vegetable oil

✓ I teaspoon medium curry powder

✓ I carton (500ml) passata (liquidised tomatoes)

✓ approx. $^1/_3$ of a 400g tin coconut milk (freeze the remainder in two batches – it can cook from frozen next time)

✓ basmati rice

Method

• Put the chopped carrots in a little water in a saucepan with the lid on and allow to boil for five minutes. In the meantime, chop the onion and chicken and add with the oil to a large frying pan or wok. As you fry the onion and chicken, add the curry powder, and leave the lid off so that it fries rather than steams.

- When the carrots are soft, liquidise them in their own water with a hand-held blender. Next, add the carrot purée, the passata and the coconut milk to the chicken mixture and stir together. Once the mixture comes to the boil, turn down the heat and allow to simmer for ten minutes until cooked.

- Add the rice to the same saucepan you used for the carrots and cover with boiling water. Once boiling, place the lid firmly on and turn off the heat. Approximately eight minutes later, drain the rice completely, return it to the saucepan and put the lid back on. To serve, simply fluff the rice with a fork for perfect basmati.

- This curry dish is best served in a bowl as it is very soupy. Kids love that about this curry. It is sweet, nutritious and not too spicy.

෨෴ℓ

So why should we put such an effort into children's fruit and vegetable consumption? To put it simply, if you sat your child down and gave him a head of broccoli to eat for starters, he would find it difficult to finish and he would certainly notice it going down.

One would be enough. He would not want another head of broccoli. He would not ask for seconds. He would have already spent enough of his time and effort biting, chewing and swallowing it. His brain would have registered this effort and acknowledged that he had eaten plenty. He would be full.

Exaggerated as this example is, the message is clear. In this head of broccoli he would have consumed folic acid, vitamin C, fibre, water and a number of nutrients, of which many are yet unnamed, that may prove beneficial to health. And he would have consumed the calorie equivalent of no more than one 'mini' bar of chocolate, if that. In short, silly as this example might seem, it represents the essence of why our kids need to consume more fruit and vegetables. Value for calories is what they represent. Vegetables are, in fact, low-calorie nutrient bombshells. They supply an array of antioxidant nutrients along with other vitamins, minerals, fibre and water. There is no vitamin pill out there that will give you the same nutrient absorption rate as that achieved by eating good old-fashioned fruit and vegetables. I have worked in the nutrition supplement industry, and this much I know. **Nothing can ever replace the goodness of real vegetables.**

We all know that we should consume more anti-oxidants, to have younger-looking skin, better heart health and to reduce our risk of developing all cancers.

We need to understand that our children are furiously building cells every day. Not only are they regenerating cells, as we do, from our skin to our insides, but they have the added burden of having to grow longer legs, stronger arms, bigger feet and heavier bones, to boot.

Children have immense requirements for nutrients as they grow and, think about it, you want them to make the best version of themselves that they can. I often explain this concept to adults as the idea of buying the biggest, most expensive car you can imagine and driving it onto the garage forecourt to get fuel. Do you put any old tractor diesel into it? No. You wait patiently, until the cleanest-looking pump, with the highest-octane fuel, becomes available, because you respect this beautiful shiny new machine and you expect to get the best performance possible from it by feeding it only the very best fuel. You can see my point, I think.

My third rule of thumb, in short, is to ask yourself every day, **HAVE THEY HAD THEIR FRUIT AND VEGETABLES TODAY?** Until the answer is a consistent 'Yes', a balanced diet has not been achieved.

How much is a portion of fruit or vegetables? A medium-sized apple, orange or pear constitutes a portion, as do two small kiwi fruit or two plums: you get the idea. In terms of vegetable portions a cup of soup or salad will do it, or three dessertspoons of any other vegetable (also measured as half a cup). When you realise what eight portions looks like on a plate, it might seem as though it will take quite an effort to get your kids to consume this much bulk. If you use my many tricks above, however, you will sail through it. The good news is that all of this consumption comes at a low calorie cost, thus ensuring that your kids' weight will return to normal, over time.

Curry in a Hurry

There are plenty of days when I need to follow my ten-minute rule: I need to have dinner on the table within ten minutes of walking through the front door, to avoid the kids snacking and complaining of hunger (more on this later).

This curry works only for those kids who already like their vegetables and their curry, so it might be something to work towards over the coming weeks. It serves about four hungry or six small kids, or, of course, two hungry parents and two small kids!

Ingredients

✓ I large onion, peeled and chopped

✓ ½ red pepper, chopped

✓ 4 chicken breasts or 6 chicken thighs, chopped

✓ 2 teaspoons medium curry powder

✓ 2 tablespoons vegetable oil

✓ I 400g tin chopped tomatoes or a 500ml carton passata

✓ frozen cauliflower

✓ frozen peas

✓ fresh coriander

✓ a pinch of salt

Method

- Place the onion, pepper, chicken, curry powder and oil in a large frying pan and cook, with the lid off, for five minutes, stirring occasionally. Next add the tomatoes and as much cauliflower as desired. Cook for a further five minutes and then add some frozen peas and a pinch of salt.

- Allow this to cook for five more minutes, then serve with fresh coriander, accompanied by rice and some toasted (perhaps from frozen) naan bread, if desired.

- In both curries in this chapter, the chicken can be replaced by chickpeas (one large can replaces two to three chicken breasts) as a vegetarian alternative. I often add some chickpeas to the mixture, along with the chicken, to vary taste and texture and also to introduce the notion of vegetarian alternatives to meat. Instead of using four chicken breasts, for instance, I might use two chicken fillets and one tin of chickpeas (drained and rinsed). Most kids love baked beans, so they will probably enjoy other cooked beans (legumes) in a tasty dish such as this.

Rule 4:

We do not need to buy organic foods

By the time I had served the last head of organic cabbage I've ever interacted with, I couldn't tell the bugs from the black pepper. My mother regularly brings me organic vegetables, potatoes, eggs and fruit from the weekly market in her west Cork town. The last organic head of cabbage she bought as a gift for me was so time-consuming to process, from washing it to drowning its many inhabitants, that I completed the task very poorly.

I love the idea of organic fresh green cabbage, covered in mud and silt and slimy little creatures, until the idea of washing it meticulously, and adding salt to a sink of water to 'clean' the tiny creatures, as I explain to my children, becomes a reality. To my mind, I have enough to do on a working day, between working for pay in the mornings and for free (parenting) in the afternoons, not to want to have to spend hours poring over every leaf of a curly green cabbage. There simply do not seem to be enough hours in the day for it. Yes, of course, organic produce is better for the planet, I utterly agree, but very often I need my cabbage presented to me in a clean, mud-and bug-free form, so that I can chop it, boil it and eat it, all in a matter of stress-free minutes.

Is it better for my kids that they get used to eating cabbage, begin to love it and now eat it regularly because I buy the pre-washed ones? Or should I only feed them the organic equivalent, which, trust me, would be a rare treat in my house, with all the work involved? For me the answer to this question is a resounding 'Yes: it is better for them just to eat cabbage, any cabbage, as long as it is clean and fresh.' They will get all the nutrients and fibre and enjoyment, give or take, from a common or garden non-organic cabbage as they would from the organic equivalent. There is not enough evidence to prove the contrary. All of my kids love cabbage, incidentally, not because they see it rarely, but because they see a little of it, often, as part of one of their favourite dinners. This is why I gently asked my mother to dispense with the organic cabbage, and now she will bring me a turnip (my poor husband) or some parsnips instead, which I simply have to peel and chop.

In an ideal world, of course, we would all have our own nice organic patch out the back, with a doe-eyed Jersey cow grazing upon it, providing us with all our seasonal fresh vegetables, fruit, organic milk and cream; and, of course, eggs and chickens from our flawless flock. In the real world, however, most of us buy our goods from supermarkets, shops and markets. This is how the world works. Some of us produce food and others buy their produce. We may dabble in growing the odd window box of herbs or trellis of tomatoes, but generally speaking we let others produce our food and we buy according to our needs. What I think we buy into when we insist that our foods are produced organically is the notion of 'clean' foods for our growing kids and also the notion of a 'sustainable' way of farming. Yes, organic farming practices are designed to encourage the conservation of soil and water and also to produce less pollution. As for cleaner food, this depends on your point of view. Those who argue against organic methods claim, for example, that the use of manure as fertiliser is not so clean when you consider its source and the reality that it can carry the *E.coli* bacteria that cause gastrointestinal illness (thus my rigorous washing of organic vegetables). Those in favour of organic produce argue that it contains significantly lower volumes of such contaminants as pesticides in fruit and vegetables, growth hormones in meats and antibiotics in chickens.

Organic yoghurt-covered rice cake, anyone?

A lot of us, as parents, however, because we cannot produce our own organic food, have recently bought into this notion of buying 'organic only' produce. We make declarations to this effect to our friends and family and thus fall prey to a growing industry that then plays on our need to be *seen* to buy the right thing for our kids when buying processed foods as well as whole foods. Organic yoghurt-covered rice cake, anyone? I'm sorry to say that little or no yoghurt is sacrificed in the making of such a product. Instead, what you feed your child in this snack, while pottering around the supermarket for instance, is an exorbitantly expensive morsel in which most calories come from sugar and saturated fat. Organic or otherwise, this is not good food. When it contains as much sugar and fat as it does, it represents 'treat' food and, as such, should be considered a once or twice weekly thing only. Your child would be far better off having an own-brand, cheap as chips, non-organically produced banana, for its fibre and nutrient content, for a fraction of the price. You will find that the yoghurt-covered rice cake is devoid of any significant amount of either fibre or nutrients.

I often refer to this concept as 'public parenting'. No judgement intended on this: I would just like to point out that because we like to be *seen* to do the right thing, and with only the best of intentions, we are susceptible to being a little ripped off by the price of organically produced foodstuffs that are unnecessary for health, which we very often buy for our kids. Our kids do not need these foods.

> Because we like to be *seen* to do the right thing we are susceptible to being a little ripped off by the price of organically produced foodstuffs that are unnecessary for health.

Processed organic foods will certainly contain fewer pesticide residues than ordinary versions, or none at all. There is no denying that these foods contain fewer food additives, such as sweeteners, artificial colours or flavours. This is a good thing. We can, though, get distracted by quality over quantity. The quality may be good, but if the quantity of fat or sugar in a product is high we still have to limit its intake by our children.

When it comes to raw fruit and vegetables and their nutrient content, many in the organic camp will show you evidence that strongly suggests that they are more nutritious. Antioxidant content in general will be shown to be higher, specifically of vitamin C, iron and calcium, as well as a host of micronutrients (those needed in very small amounts). Equally, they will claim that their organic produce has a higher content of phytochemicals (chemicals found naturally in plants) that are of great benefit to our health. The answer is not clear yet, however, as to whether organic produce is *actually* higher in antioxidant and nutrient levels than that produced non-organically. Experiments (regarding freshness of foodstuffs, for instance) have not been repeated often enough to be considered solid evidence of this.

For the moment, therefore, nutrient content is, broadly speaking, comparable in both types of produce. There is no conclusive evidence to the contrary. In the real world, the level of antioxidants your child gets from a fresh green head of broccoli are adequate as long as it has not been boiled to a pulp! Colour in nature equals antioxidants. The more colour and crunch your child gets on a regular daily basis, the better (within reason: we do not need to eat exclusively raw foods). Non-organically produced fruit and vegetables will give your child the same amount of iron as the organically produced versions and certainly the same amount of fibre, bulk and chewing effort involved in ingestion. If you wash the 'clean' broccoli with as much vigour as you would the muddy version, you will reduce the amount of pesticide residue in it. In other words, you do the best you can.

I also draw the line at buying organic chocolate at five times the price of the non-organic equivalent. I recommend to clients, when they really want chocolate, to go out and buy just that, chocolate, not some wafer-containing bar, but the real thing. They will often come back with the idea of buying organic dark chocolate at a premium price I would never recommend. Yes, by all means buy the expensive one if you can afford to do so, but I will guarantee that your kids will not like it, and neither will you, unless you have an evolved palate that can enjoy a very dark, thus slightly bitter chocolate. Most of us, and certainly our kids, prefer a milkier chocolate: therefore, if you buy small, good-quality bars (Animal Bars are our favourite) you are keeping your eye more closely on the message, which is that 'a little of what you fancy does you good'. Eating what you, or your kids, do not like really serves no purpose, in my opinion. We will first eat the dark one that we did not really want, and then go in search of the milk version! **Quantity and**

quality are two separate things. We need to spot that on behalf of our kids.

One of the biggest misconceptions about eating healthily is that good food costs lots of money. This is one of the primary excuses we use for buying cheap oven chips, chicken Kiev, fish fingers, potato waffles, biscuits, multi-packs of chocolate wafer bars, fruit juices and the like. We theorise that buying potatoes, chicken fillets, fish, meat, new season baby potatoes, berries, fruit and fresh vegetables is prohibitively expensive and that we have no hope of being able to afford to buy them all the time for our family. Who can afford such luxuries as eating whole fresh foods every day of the week? My answer to this is simple. You can. We all can. How? By shopping wisely. We do not need to buy organic *super-foods* in order to achieve a balanced diet for our family. We simply need to buy as many *whole* foods as possible, as cheaply as possible, so as to prove to ourselves that it is in fact more economical to live this way. Variety is certainly the spice of life when it comes to food. By 'whole foods' I mean just that: foods that are still in their whole state. Choose potatoes, not chips. Buy porridge oats, not oat flakes. Buy apples, not apple juice.

I usually shop twice a week. The first time might be on a Monday morning when I go to my local branch of a very cheap supermarket chain and start my shopping with whatever fruit and vegetables are on offer that day. If kiwis and grapes are the least expensive today, guess what fruit the children will get in their lunchboxes that week. When a pineapple is being almost given away for free I buy the thing. I top it, tail it, take the skin off, cut it into quarters, take out the woody stem from each quarter and chop the remainder into bite-sized pieces. If I put it on the counter-top in my kitchen at after-school snack time it will not last twenty minutes. The beauty of buying one at such a price is that it has to be eaten now. It is often so ripe that it is only a couple of days away from the rotting stage in its development. That is why it is on offer in the first place.

A lot of us believe that our kids will not eat fruit. You may have good reason to believe this. Most of the fruit we get is not ripened on the tree, unlike in Mediterranean countries, for instance, where fruit goes from field to plate in a couple of days. Much of our fruit is imported rock-hard and subsequently ripened in a shed at the port where it landed. Ethylene gas is used to ripen bananas, for example, that arrive on our shores as green as the grass in your garden. If you have ever tasted a banana in Thailand, by comparison, you will remember that it was lumpy, bumpy, yellow and brown and smelled and tasted more like a banana-flavoured children's sweet than the kind of bananas we are used to here: in fact, utterly fabulous. So I agree – much of our fruit leaves a lot to be desired when it comes to taste and freshness. I can agree that an organic apple off a tree in your own garden tastes infinitely better than a shop-bought, perfectly red one. However, if you use a bit of wisdom and knowledge when you shop you can get the best available fruit for the price best suited to your pocket. Organic fruit is often sold at a reduced price and tastes great then because it is being sold at its peak of ripeness.

So when our kids decide not to like fruit, we could introduce them to the array of cheap alternatives to the perfect-looking but often tasteless apple. Let them try cheap and cheerful bananas (rather than the perfect organic fun-sized one); present them with a fruit salad (on a day when you have the time to make it) containing cheap kiwis, grapes, apple, banana, mandarin and a squeeze of lemon or orange juice (to prevent everything going brown). Why not try fruit cocktail from a tin for a change? (Pour the juice down the sink; it is just sugared water.) Frozen berries are a lot cheaper than fresh when the fresh berries are out of season. It is a fantastic idea to have a stash of frozen berries ready to be thawed out in a matter of minutes on the counter-top (or seconds in the microwave) and served with custard (home-made or a store cupboard version).

Baby Banana Muffins

Some time ago I purchased a non-stick bite-sized-muffin tin that can bake twenty-four muffins at once. I had grown tired of using tiny paper cases that invariably got squished as my little ones got hold of them to play 'baking' with their teddies. So I gave up buying them and missed always having a stash of frozen bite-sized muffins in my freezer, handy for both lunch-boxes and for when anyone called unexpectedly (they thaw out in mere minutes).

Once I purchased my wonder tin, I next discovered the joys of spray oil. Having steered well clear of anything that promised a one-calorie spray, for the sheer daftness of the concept, I suddenly realised that using this spray meant I could dispense altogether with using paper cases for either tiny or large muffins. So I bought non-stick large muffin tins too, along with a two-pound loaf tin (to be used in a later recipe for brown bread).

Ingredients

✓ 3 very ripe bananas

✓ 150g wholemeal flour

✓ 50g white flour

✓ 150g brown sugar

✓ 1½ teaspoons baking powder

✓ 125ml (½ cup) vegetable oil

✓ 4 tablespoons plain yoghurt (vanilla yoghurt or any left-over yoghurt will do)

✓ 1 teaspoon vanilla extract

✓ a small pinch of salt

✓ spray vegetable oil (just for ease and speed, though feel free
   to use butter)

Method

- Get someone small to mash the bananas for you on a plate.
  Put all the dry ingredients into a bowl and combine. Put the
  oil, yoghurt and vanilla extract into a separate container and
  mix with a fork or whisk.

- Add the mashed banana to the wet ingredients and stir
  before pouring into the dry mixture. Stir the entire mixture
  with a fork, as little as possible, until just combined, as this
  makes the fluffiest muffins. Finally, liberally spray the muffin
  tin with the oil, then put tiny spoonfuls of the mixture into
  each case, leaving room for them to rise. You could make
  some bigger muffins with the remaining mixture.

- Bake in a pre-heated oven at 180°C for approximately
  twelve minutes for small muffins and approximately
  eighteen minutes for large ones. When they have cooled,
  freeze a batch to have on stand-by. It is always a good idea
  to freeze extra cakes, otherwise they get eaten!

ৼৡ

Is it better to limit yourself to buying only organic, thus expensive, food for your kids, which they may or may not eat, or to buy an array of cheaper fruit and vegetables to broaden your kids' food horizons and encourage them to constantly try new tastes? When we aim for perfection I believe we are doomed to failure. If we could attain dietary perfection, life could be perfect. It is not. Instead, **if we buy whole foods, in as wide a variety as takes our interest, we will do very well indeed, from a nutritional standpoint.** There are not so many more benefits to organic produce that it is worth limiting our kids to what they may or may not like of them. Is it better that they eat some cheap sugar-snap peas than nothing green that day? Yes.

Seasonal food tends to be much better value than the imported equivalent. Because of a surplus in supply, apples that are falling off the trees during the month of October are at their cheapest and are the best-tasting apples of the year. Get your kids to eat them until they come out of their ears! Apples in the lunch box, stewed apple with ice cream or custard for dessert, apple sauce with pork, apple slices with cheese as an afternoon snack, apples chopped into cereal in the morning. Then the day will come when your child has had enough of apples. Great, the season is over and now frozen berries are inexpensive. The reason we gave fresh berries to our kids all summer is that they were being sold for as little as they will ever be. So all summer long your children had berries on their cereal, berry smoothies for afternoon snack, berries and custard or ice cream for dessert or, occasionally, home-made berry crumble. The same applies to vegetables: keep food varied and interesting by buying the bargains.

On my second shopping trip of the week I will go to the better-stocked mainstream supermarket where my bargains will include less common fruits and vegetables, more varieties of lettuce, long-stemmed broccoli or the purple-sprouting variety as well as such whole foods as tinned beans ('naked' versions as well as those in tomato sauce), yoghurts and cheeses, baking and general cooking ingredients. As often as not, I do this shop online earlier in the week, in the comfort of my home, so as to free up time in my working week. Again, own-brand whole foods in these supermarkets can be very inexpensive. Trust me, I can tell no difference – apart from the price – between an own-brand tin of chopped tomatoes and a branded one. My kids will benefit just as much from me making my own tomato sauce (in minutes) to accompany that evening's chicken casserole as they would if it had cost twice the price. What they will benefit from is eating little or no processed food in their day. They will have had home-made sauce that took seconds to make, with none of the additives found in tomato sauce from a jar.

Our kids do not need expensive processed food. They benefit more from unadulterated (inexpensive) whole foods that are simply assembled into a tasty meal. Instead of potato waffles, which are full of salt and fat, give your child chopped potatoes fried in a little olive oil (which has proven health benefits). Instead of chicken Kiev, give your child a chicken breast or thigh (a cheaper alternative) with red pesto on top baked in the oven in less time than it takes to heat the Kiev. In place of oven chips, put baby potatoes in the oven for exactly the same length of time, drizzled with olive oil and maybe some herbes de Provence. To replace fish fingers, brush frozen white fish with beaten egg and coat with crushed cornflakes or oats (your kids will love crushing the cornflakes, incidentally) and bake in the oven with olive oil for the same length of time as it would take to cook fish fingers. Buy good food cheaply: it can cost a fraction of the price of processed food, and it will take no longer to prepare. It is, in my estimation, significantly better that most of your kids' food is home-made instead of pre-packaged, even if the pre-packaged food is organic. I have a 'nine out of ten' rule when it comes to this principle in my house. Food is home-made nine times out of ten, not always. My kids also get fish fingers and beans for tea when necessary, believe me.

Fun and Tasty Chicken or Fish Goujons

Most kids love fish fingers. Most kids love chicken goujons. While I might cook the odd fish finger (which is half fish and half a poor-quality high-fat bread covering), because the kids would feel 'weird' if they were never allowed to eat them, I tend to draw the line at shop-bought frozen chicken goujons. You will notice that no quality statements are ever made about the chicken or other ingredients used and I'm afraid I always think 'noses and toes' when I think about the mechanically reclaimed 'meat' so often used in these products. Squeamish as I may sound, I do think I can do better than that for my kids. I can guarantee yours will love these as much as any shop-bought equivalent and minimal effort is needed to make them. This recipe serves four hungry or six small kids.

Ingredients

✓ 3 chicken breasts or 3 large fillets of firm white fish (such as haddock)

✓ I egg, beaten with a little milk

✓ I cup approx. crushed cornflakes or oats

✓ 2 tablespoons of olive oil

Method

• Cut the chicken or fish into long strips (or shorter strips for small kids). Place in a bowl with the egg and milk mixture and stir around to coat completely. Leave to sit in the egg mixture while you organise the other ingredients.

- Crush the cornflakes, if using (with a rolling pin, in a plastic bag) and spread them (or the oats) over a flat plate. Pour the oil into a wide-based frying pan and turn on the heat. Take the chicken or fish from the egg mixture and roll in the oats or flakes and then put them in the oil. Repeat until the pan contains enough goujons to allow them all to fry at high heat. Do not be tempted to over-crowd the pan as the mixture will boil!

- If you need to keep them warm while finishing off, put them in a warm oven for a few minutes. In fact, most kids prefer these not too hot.

- These are best served with ketchup, peas, broccoli and potato wedges.

৩৽৵

Potato Wedges

This is so easy!

Rooster potatoes are great 'all-rounders' when it comes to needing a convenient spud. I buy mine pre-washed. All you have to do is cut each potato first in half (lengthwise), then each half into halves, then each quarter into eighths (if big enough). Place on a baking tray and drizzle with some olive oil, a hint of salt and pepper and my favourite quick-fix flavour, herbes de Provence (thyme works well too). Bake at 180°C for approximately 45 minutes.

∽∾

We've discussed fruit and vegetables, but we can also tend to think that only organic meat is nutritious. I would argue that we can be a little off the point here too. An organic sausage will have as little 'meat' in it as a non-organically produced sausage and is thus about as non-nutritious as its non-organically produced cousin. Yes, organic beef will be free from hormones, and that is worth paying for, if you can afford it. I often buy lamb instead of beef to make a shepherd's pie or mince and rice, or indeed burgers, because lamb, by definition, is not intensively reared (it does not live long enough to have to be). Instead, it tends to live a short but happy life up on a hill, somewhere green and

mountainous, with its flock. As such, it will be free
from the myriad components found in today's
intensively farmed beef. Lamb steaks represent good
value when compared to tiny chops, as we get to eat
the entire thing, and of course shoulder of lamb is
perfect for a curry or tagine (which kids love because
of its sweetness). Lamb is certainly a lot cheaper than
organically produced beef.

Buying chicken can be a minefield when choosing
the best version for your family. Your child does not
benefit from eating only organic chicken. At four
times the price of non-organic chicken, I find it hard
to justify buying it. If you can get 'antibiotic-free'
chicken at a reasonable price I would recommend
that. But do not be fooled, however, into thinking
that this lucky chicken was allowed to roam free and
was therefore not dosed with antibiotics. It will have
been. But 'antibiotic-free' chicken is not given
antibiotics just before slaughter, so the flesh, by the
time you purchase it, is free of antibiotics – and
better for your family. If and when I buy an organic
chicken it is because it is on sale (in other words, it
has to be eaten today or tomorrow). When the
chicken is eaten, I boil the bones for two hours (like
my mother always did). I make a lovely chicken stock
from these organic bones and use it to make the next
soup or stew. This might sound labour-intensive, but
it is not: bones, water and heat are the only

components. There is no effort on my part. It is great fun to get one of your kids to lift the lid off this concoction as it boils, by the way, if you ever try it. It utterly horrifies them. As for the visiting play-date child, the fun is endless! If you wish to buy corn-fed chicken, it is taste you are chasing; if you wish to buy free-range it is more an issue of humane production. Again, do not be fooled into thinking that these fortunate chicks spent their lives frolicking around a farmyard. For the most part (in other words the mass-produced versions) these beasts were reared in a shed, intensively, for a short few weeks, with a couple of square feet to move around in, rather than caged, and that is it. They are still given antibiotics: they still do not roam free. When they genuinely roam about a farmyard and are allowed to live longer, lovelier lives you will notice the price difference. My point here is that you should buy whatever you can afford. Whatever type of chicken you buy, from a nutritional perspective your kids will benefit more from having a home-made chicken dinner instead of frozen chicken goujons.

Equally, organic milk may contain fewer chemical contaminants than non-organic milk, but when you go through three litres a day, as we do in my house, you tend to buy the regular stuff. I think it is important to strike a balance that suits your children's needs, as well as your pocket.

My rule number four is **WE DO NOT NEED TO BUY ORGANIC FOODS** to feed our kids well. A desire for perfection in food is a barrier to success: it sets us up for failure. The middle ground is more my territory when it comes to food: first aim to do your best and then aim to do so consistently. The reason that I do not buy organically produced milk, for example, is that it is too expensive to justify at present, and my kids consume so much of it that any taste difference between the organic and non-organic versions is of no significance to my family.

When it comes to carrots, however, I do buy only organic. Why? Put chopped-up carrot of both types on a plate on your counter-top at snack time and do the taste test. My money is on your kids eating all the organic carrots, and little or none of the other. I have tried this and the taste difference is so significant that there will always be a clear winner. I am, therefore, inclined to agree that organic fruit and vegetables taste better. There are also likely to be fewer organo-phosphates (pesticides) in organic produce, and these are linked to cancer risk; but there is currently no evidence strong enough to suggest that any extra health benefits can be gained from eating only organic foods. They might taste better, but nutrient quantity is largely the same.

Rule 5:

If you can name it, you can consider it

I t was Hippocrates, the father of medicine, who said in the fourth century BC, 'Let food be thy medicine and medicine be thy food.' **Our kids do not need special or functional foods.** Good foods – by which I mean whole foods – already fulfil our children's nutritional needs. Food supplies our children with energy to grow, play and learn. Food also acts as a source of fibre, water and the myriad nutrients that are needed to repair and build tissue and carry out metabolic processes. So a good-quality diet can give your child all they need to grow up strong, bright and thriving.

Why, then, is the purchase of 'functional' foods one of the biggest growth areas in the US (and, indeed, western) food industry? Functional foods are claimed to offer us additional benefits to those of ordinary foods that may reduce the risk of disease, in general terms, while also promoting optimal health. Clearly we need to sit up and take notice of these foods, you would think. It would be remiss of us not to feed our kids bucket-loads of these foods. We want to give our kids every advantage, I think you will agree. However, I do not buy these foods and I do not feed these foods to my children.

'Functional' foods have become very trendy of late. What are they, exactly, and where do we get them? They include yoghurt drinks that contain probiotics; cereal bars that contain prebiotics; spreads for our bread that contain plant sterols. They also include the likes of food supplements, such as garlic extract, that are taken on their own, separately from food. This moves us into the branch of an enormous growth industry called 'neutraceuticals'.

Let me give a brief overview. Functional foods first appeared in Japan in the 1980s. They are described, by the American Dietetic Association for instance, as foods – including whole foods and fortified and enriched or enhanced foods – that have a potentially beneficial effect on health when consumed as part of a varied diet on a regular basis at effective levels. This means, essentially, a food to which a new ingredient (or, in many cases, more of an existing ingredient) is added, thereby giving the 'improved' food new qualities. Because this new and improved food now contains what are termed 'bioactive' compounds it may be advertised on the basis that it reduces the risk of chronic disease beyond basic nutritional function and can therefore improve health.

What surprises most people, when I discuss this topic with them, is the fact that many of our common or garden foods are already potent sources of these bioactive compounds. For example, tomatoes are the best source of lycopene, considered to be one of nature's most potent antioxidants. When you cook tomatoes they appear to release more of their lycopene content for absorption and even tomato purée, tomato sauces and tinned tomatoes give us mighty doses of this powerful antioxidant. Compounds in broccoli (and other cruciferous vegetables, such as cauliflower) have been shown to reduce the risk of getting certain cancers, when consumed regularly. (I often add broccoli to curries, as it soaks up all the flavour of the curry and is then consumed in large quantities.) Citrus fruits (lemons, grapefruit and oranges) contain substances called limonoids that can reduce the risk of cancer, as might regular consumption (five to six cups a day) of green tea (now *that* my kids will not drink – yet!). We are all aware of the benefits of omega-3 fatty acids in reducing the risk of developing cardiovascular disease, one of our primary killers in the West, which we can get from both oily fish and flax seed; and flax seed has also been shown to reduce the risk of certain cancers, as has soy bean consumption. The humble oat (from that daily bowl of porridge or on top of stewed apple, as a crumble) can dramatically reduce blood cholesterol levels.

The nutraceuticals section of the functional food industry involves extracting bioactive components of food, such as the active part of garlic, or the flavonoid part of red grapes (known to benefit heart health when consumed regularly in red wine). These specific components of foods are extracted and sold as supplements in concentrated form. Thus, garlic supplements containing concentrated allicin (the active ingredient in garlic) have been shown in studies to reduce blood cholesterol, high blood pressure and the risk of developing some cancers. Equally, cranberry juice has been shown to lower the incidence of urinary tract infections, and it can now be found in capsule form, as can an array of other neutraceuticals. Even beef, the often maligned source of good-quality protein and readily absorbed iron, has recently been shown to contain a very impressive bioactive compound called CLA (conjugated linoleic acid) in the fat on the meat! It is now hoped that its content in milk can be increased, thereby providing some protection against certain cancers and promoting weight loss. Amazing! Think of all the times you have discarded the fat on the meat.

What are probiotics and prebiotics? Approximately four hundred species of bacteria inhabit our gut (gastrointestinal system). They fall into two broad categories: those that are beneficial and those that are detrimental to our gastrointestinal health. Of the beneficial bugs in our system, lactic acid bacteria are the ones that have attracted most attention. These so-called 'good' bacteria are found in fermented dairy products (e.g. yoghurt) and are known as probiotics.

These good bacteria are found to improve intestinal balance and, as a result, enhance our digestive health, reducing bloating and constipation and increasing our immunity to some pathogenic bacteria ('bad' bugs). In short, probiotics are bacteria of the species that normally exist in our gut, which are put into a product so that it can be named 'live' or 'bio'. In theory, these so-called 'good' bacteria can withstand the acid in our stomach and reach our intestine, where they can colonise it and grow, to do us some good. The good, really, is a matter of displacement, a territorial battle against the 'bad' bacteria. If you have copious quantities of 'good' bacteria around, there will not be as much room for the 'bad' bacteria to grow. The 'good' bacteria can help our immune system and fight a range of infections, so they should be taken seriously.

When buying yoghurts, therefore, I do buy 'live'/'bio' yoghurts, but I stay away from the over-sweetened, watered-down drinking yoghurt that comes – far too conveniently – in bottles or cartons. The reason is that I strongly believe we should sit down to eat (see Rule 2). Our kids should consume yoghurt, which has been around for centuries, in as whole-food a manner as possible, by which I mean it should have a short ingredients list, and be eaten with a spoon while sitting at a table or counter-top or indeed a school desk.

A good-quality yoghurt, either 'full-fat' or 'low-fat', contains milk, sugar and fruit (if it is a fruit yoghurt), the lactobacteria we have discussed and a great big full stop at the end of the list. Nothing more needs to be present in our yoghurts. If the ingredients list is as long as your child's arm, in a product that should be very straightforward to make, for me it represents a poor-quality product. I do not wish to feed my kids acidity regulators (such as sodium citrate), fructose-glucose syrup, sweeteners (aspartame, acesulfame K) or emulsifiers such as acetic acid esters of mono and diglycerides of fatty acids. When a product reads like a chemistry set, I move to the next one on the shelf.

> I do not wish to feed my kids acidity regulators (such as sodium citrate), fructose-glucose syrup, sweeteners (aspartame, acesulfame K) or emulsifiers such as acetic acid esters of mono and diglycerides of fatty acids. When a product reads like a chemistry set, I move to the next one on the shelf.

In addition to probiotics are the foods that they feed upon, called prebiotics. The prebiotics that the good bugs grow on are substances such as fibre, sugars and carbohydrates. Thus, prebiotics, which promote the growth of good bacteria, are another functional component of interest to nutritional scientists and can, when consumed regularly, help promote the health of our gut. Such bioactive compounds are found in foods such as artichokes and bananas.

With the best of intentions in mind, we buy extraordinary amounts of yoghurt drinks on the back of the marketing of so-called 'good' bacteria. We want to give our kids only the best and we want it in a convenient, mess-free packaging. And, best of all, our kids love drinking these products. Scientific opinion, however, is divided on whether or not they are truly beneficial or necessary for health. Whether the 'good' bacteria survive in any significant number and get to their destination is still up for debate. Nonetheless, you may think, they certainly won't do our kids any harm.

Or will they?

I will never have these yoghurt drinks in the fridge, or indeed lunchboxes. Why? Because, when they are marketed to kids, they are always brim-full of sugar. It is assumed that kids only want sweet. Yes, if this is all they are ever given. (The 'adult' versions often contain a sugar alternative, which is much worse, in my opinion.) These yoghurt drinks are rotting our children's teeth: every day a considerable amount of sugar is left sitting on the teeth of children, who often consume them during their morning break at school. The harm that this consistent hit of sugar can do from both a calorie and dental health perspective far outweighs any possible good these products might do, in my opinion. Instead, my kids get old-fashioned yoghurts in their lunch boxes and they also get a spoon (or medicine spoon when the dishwasher is full). One or two of them will even have plain full-fat yoghurt with fruit as a dessert in the afternoon, with no added sugar. The full-fat version seems so creamy that they do not notice its lack of excess sweetness. Of course milk is already sweet because it contains a sugar called lactose.

I always buy good-quality plain and fruit yoghurts, both full-fat and low-fat. They are inexpensive and have a texture that kids love. A naturally set full-fat yoghurt can seem luxurious. Ordinary full-fat yoghurts (those that are not 'Greek' style, or 'custard' style) are naturally low in fat. Milk comes out of a cow at about 3.5% fat, so ordinary full-fat yoghurt remains at about 3.5% fat. In other words, it is already a low-fat product. Children often like lower-fat alternatives too. In these products the cream has simply been removed, as in the low-fat milk in your fridge. However, I never buy 'fat-free' or 'diet' yoghurts as they tend to contain starches and thickeners and, often, artificial sweeteners. There is such a variety of yoghurt available that it's impossible to expect your child to like all of them. Experiment! My six-year-old loves full-fat plain yoghurt best, while my eight-year-old loves low-fat raspberry. My ten-year-old consumes yoghurt only as part of dessert and wouldn't be caught dead choosing yoghurt as a stand-alone snack!

Why should children eat yoghurts in the first place? The answer is that yoghurts are a great source of calcium and protein. Our children can go through extraordinary growth spurts, never more so than as teenagers. They need a daily supply of calcium to maximise bone density during such periods of growth. This is a golden opportunity that should not be overlooked. By the age of eighteen our children will have laid down up to eighty-five or even ninety per cent of their bone mass. If we set up good habits from a very early age, our kids will reach for yoghurt at snack time as readily as for a piece of fruit.

As all yoghurts contain beneficial bacteria, by definition they are a 'cultured' product; you can rest assured that you are giving your child something that they need. Many of our yoghurts today are called 'live-bio' yoghurts without having to be the expensive bottled drink version and they still contain the beneficial bacteria. I would much rather see my children eat food with a spoon than knock it back as a drink. Ideally our kids eat only at the table, and yoghurt is part of a meal or a planned snack: it is not a drink consumed in passing, en route from A to B, just because you saw it in the fridge and fancied it. **This is called 'passive consumption' of calories and it is what we wish to avoid at all costs.** We need our children to start getting a lot more value per calorie if we want to get their weight back under control.

As for sugar-free products, I will certainly not feed these to my kids. These products might promise 'low calories' but they contain what are, to my mind, toxins for a growing body. A child's kidneys, liver and bladder are still growing. They can certainly do without added toxins, which it is the job of these organs to remove. If they were not removed, these ingredients would prove toxic. As an adult, perhaps the occasional sugar-free product can be consumed. Our organs have fully developed and grown, but our kids' organs have not. **Children do not benefit in any way from artificial sweeteners.**

Our children need to eat good-quality (and often inexpensive) foods such as fruit, vegetables, whole grains, yoghurts and meat, eggs or fish. Healthy, growing kids really have no added need for special, or functional, ingredients. Concentrate on what they are eating (not on what they are avoiding) when making your shopping list, and keep it simple. Many new products, from cereals to cereal bars, contain prebiotics, in a bid to get us to buy them rather than the competing products. Do we benefit from them? Yes, but they are already in plentiful supply in such foods as bananas, onions and honey (honey goes beautifully on porridge). They include complex carbohydrates that are found in whole grains, for instance. The theory is that they will help to grow the

KILKENNY COUNTY LIBRARY

bacteria that we require and so are even of greater benefit to us than probiotics. This theory may stand up to scrutiny over time. But I feel our diet already supplies these components aplenty, when we eat the right foods. Therefore, I do not look for them as ingredients in processed foods.

What *do* I buy? Research has shown, over the years and years spent investigating dietary habits around the world, that those who consume a primarily vegetable-based diet suffer the fewest cancers. Eating a diet rich in plant foods (whole grains as well as fruit and vegetables) protects against cancer and other chronic diseases, such as cardiovascular disease and type 2 diabetes. This does not mean that your children have to become vegetarian. What it does mean is that they need to get into the habit of frequently eating plant-based foods. Not occasionally. **They need to eat fruit, vegetables and whole grains every day.** For this reason my fridge and cupboards are full of the original of the species when it comes to sources of such bioactive components.

Yoghurt (good-quality, perhaps low-fat, perhaps full-fat plain or fruit-based) supplies all the bioactive bugs my kids need. Butter gives them enough animal fats to do them good. Oily fish, a couple of times a week, supplies them with enough omega-3 fatty acids to get such jobs done as making anti-inflammatory substances in the body and regulating hormone production. I feel like a tomato 'pusher' from day one when I get my kids to try tomatoes, raw and cooked, in sauces and soups. Lycopene is an unbeatable antioxidant that should keep them alive and well for a very long time, protecting them from the ravages of time, both internally and externally. Garlic is used on a near-daily basis in my house; oats, whether milled, in instant cereal form, porridge, muesli or crumble, also feature.

As for spreads containing plant sterols, these will not be found in my house. Children start laying down cholesterol in their arteries from about the age of three. To avoid excessive cholesterol deposits I feed my children oats, beans, garlic, red grapes, apples, oily fish and olive oil, all of which have been proven through extensive research to lower overall cholesterol levels. Equally I get them to exercise (to play, for the most part), which has a proven effect on lowering blood cholesterol. I see no purpose to their consuming plant stanol esters (sterols) in any form other than certain plant foods.

To put it as simply as possible, my take on the evidence of the benefits of such functional foods is that **it is more important that you pay attention to what your kids eat than what they do not eat.** What I mean by this is that, as adults, we spend so much effort avoiding so-called 'bad' foods, from chocolates to fried foods. Then we feel that we should also include special (functional) foods as a sort of insurance policy approach to our dietary health. Instead, I feel we should turn our attention to the opposite end of the spectrum and pay close attention to what it is that is passing our kids' lips on a regular daily basis.

Three-minute Tomato Sauce

This speedy sauce goes wonderfully on pasta, chicken, white fish or pizza. I tend to make a large amount at a time (enough for two dinners at least) so that I can freeze some or have some in the fridge to help another night's cooking along. The reason I use passata in place of chopped tomatoes is that my kids will not always eat the 'bits'. This can vary according to your taste. It takes no more than three minutes on your part. I am not joking: time it! The cooker does the rest.

Ingredients

- ✓ 2 tablespoons olive oil
- ✓ I clove of garlic, peeled and chopped: this is the only hard labour involved!
- ✓ I carton (500ml) passata or I 400g tin chopped tomatoes
- ✓ a squeeze of tomato purée
- ✓ ½ teaspoon sugar
- ✓ a pinch of salt
- ✓ lots of dried oregano

Method

- Pour the olive oil into a saucepan and add the chopped garlic. Fry gently for no more than a minute; do not allow it to burn.

- Next, add the tomato passata (or chopped tomatoes), tomato purée, sugar, salt and plenty of dried oregano. Put the lid on (if you want to avoid splashes) and allow to simmer for anything from five to fifteen minutes, depending on how thick you like your sauce and how much time you have. It tastes lovely after even five short minutes. Your work, though, is done in less than three. I hope you timed it!

❧❧

My shopping list has a particular order. And yes, I do recognise how neurotic this sounds. As far as I am concerned, order is what success is all about when it comes to balanced eating. If your shopping list has an order to it that enables you to very simply plan a week's balanced eating for your family, that to me represents a plan for success. If your shopping list looks balanced, your shopping trolley will look balanced (you will be very proud of it at the check-out), your cupboards and fridge will look balanced and, you guessed it, your breakfast, lunch and dinner plates will look balanced. It is that easy. No more chaos, only order around food from now on, with my wonder list in tow. And, yes, I make lists for everything: you have probably guessed that by now. Lists save time. If you follow your list to the letter, you will not forget an essential ingredient, such as the onions without which a curry would be very sad and sorry. We do not need to spend our lives running in and out of shops: in my opinion we need to stay out of shops as far as possible.

My magic list will help you to shop as infrequently as possible, which will free up all those half-hours that you might currently spend popping to the shop nearly every day. Incidentally, if you follow my list method of shopping I can guarantee you huge savings on your weekly shop. The list is not prescriptive: it is entirely up to you to buy whatever you fancy. I'm simply offering a system for buying your foods, with ease and balance in mind. From today, I hope you will follow my lead and always shop according to food groups.

Magic shopping list

Fruit	bag of apples, mandarin oranges, grapes, pineapple, bananas, berries, raisins, kiwis, tinned grapefruit, frozen berries
Vegetables	broccoli, carrots, onions, garlic, ginger, tomatoes, butternut squash, beetroot, rocket, spring onions, peppers, avocados, frozen green beans, frozen peas
Starches	potatoes, sweet potatoes, rice, noodles, pasta, soda bread, wraps, bagels, porridge oats, bran flakes, shredded wheat, muesli
Meat, fish, other proteins	minced steak, chopped lamb shoulder, salmon, sardines (tin), whole chicken, chicken thighs, chickpeas, kidney beans
Dairy	low-fat milk, plain and fruit yoghurts, block of Cheddar, sliced Edam, mozzarella, feta, goat's cheese spread
Snacks	whole peanuts in the shell, popcorn, whole pistachios, small chocolate bars, boxes of raisins
Fats and other	olive oil, grape oil, honey and mustard dressing, caramelised onion jam, honey, butter, crunchy peanut butter, chocolate spread, wholemeal flour, cocoa powder, red pesto, green pesto, sweet chilli sauce
Household	cleaning materials, etc.

This list represents a recent shop of mine, the details of which are not as important as the principle involved. You will notice that fruit comes first in my mind. Keep it varied and inexpensive. Allow your kids to get involved in making the shopping list, for example ask them, 'What fruit would you like this week?', then buy that fruit along with others.

The vegetable list should always include greens as well as yellow/orange vegetables to ensure adequate nutrition. Frozen vegetables are a regular feature of my list.

I give my kids a source of protein every day, which might be eggs, meat, fish or vegetarian alternatives. I give them red meat, white meat, fish and legumes (such as chickpeas in a curry and kidney beans in a chilli). I find that tinned beans are very convenient to have in the store cupboard.

Dairy products include milk, yoghurt, and an array of cheeses, again to keep things interesting. Kids will not like goat's cheese, I can almost guarantee it. However, if you toast a little soda bread, spread it with a mild goat's cheese spread and top with caramelised onion relish you will be surprised by how open older children can be to the offering.

Every list should contain a 'snacks' category. We need tasty snacks in the house. Equally our kids need to get some fat, so I buy butter, nuts and chocolate weekly. The rest is easy. Try out your own list. It is fun to do, easy to execute and very thrifty in its approach.

We need to ensure that our kids get a largely plant-based diet for health, and then we won't need to worry about them having to avoid chocolate and fried foods. When your kids' habits are up and running with respect to good dietary balance, you can allow them chocolate and fried foods in moderation and regularly, as long as this happens to a plan and is not overly ad hoc.

What I believe we will teach our kids, if we allow them to buy into the notion of eating functional foods, is a future of eating poorly and 'fixing' any resulting problem (high cholesterol, say) by adding an appropriate functional food element to their diet. This is one step away from the 'pill' mentality that many of us already suffer from as adults. I also think that our children, if they are healthy and well, will benefit far more from a consistent approach to getting a largely plant-based diet past their lips than they will from using 'special' (functional) foods to take care of any nutritional deficit caused by eating too much processed food.

My rule number five is: **IF YOU CAN NAME IT, YOU CAN CONSIDER IT.** Can you list the ingredients in your child's favourite snack food? All of them? My guess is probably not. In a good-quality yoghurt there should be a short ingredients list, such as: milk; the cultures that make it a yoghurt; and perhaps a live 'bio' culture such as *Lactobacillus acidophilus*. That's two or possibly three ingredients. You can name them in a flash and that is generally a good sign that you are getting a quality product. It is what it is! If your child prefers a fruit yoghurt, the list has perhaps three additions: sugar, fruit and natural flavour. When an ingredients list in what should be a simple product is as long as your arm – which is often the case in fat-free products – this is generally not a sign of good quality. Feed your children products whose ingredients you can list off the top off your head. If you can name it, you can consider it! Since when have we needed diacetyl esters of fatty acids, for instance, in our desserts? I can't find them in my kitchen; so I tend to stay away from them in packaged form too.

You might notice that I think it is quite appropriate to give my children yoghurts containing lots of sugar. Now and again we do need sugar, for energy. The difference is that I do not give them a sugary yoghurt drink to take to school every day that will be consumed at their first break time. They have sugary yoghurt as a planned snack, with fruit, in the afternoon, or for dessert after dinner. This means that the sugar is not sitting on their teeth all day, having been consumed at ten-thirty in the morning. And they will have eaten it with a spoon, as part of a meal or as a snack, and therefore they will register that they have eaten it.

Cute Carrot and Seed Mini-Muffins

This recipe calls for a long list of ingredients, but all of these will already be sitting in your store cupboards – or will be very soon! The method, once again, is very easy. To my surprise I found that this is a great way of introducing children to eating seeds in breads. (I only added them on the off-chance that they might suit the tastebuds of one or two of my kids, but in fact they all like them, sometimes!)

Ingredients

✓ 150g wholemeal flour

✓ 50g white flour

✓ 30g sugar

✓ 50ml honey or maple syrup

✓ 125ml (½ cup) vegetable oil

✓ 2 eggs

✓ 1 teaspoon vanilla extract

✓ 1 teaspoon baking powder

✓ a small pinch of salt

✓ ¼ teaspoon mixed spice

✓ 150g grated carrot

✓ 1 tablespoon unsalted mixed seeds (I mix my own, using sesame seeds, pumpkin seeds and linseed)

Method

- As in the previous muffin recipe, you (or perhaps your little one) simply mix the dry ingredients in one bowl and the wet in another, and then combine them, stirring as little as possible. Bake them at 180°C: mini-muffins take about 12 minutes and larger ones about 18 minutes.

෴

Let food be your kids' medicine. If they eat only good-quality whole foods for the most part, their sugar intake will be under control. Functional foods have no essential role in good nutrition. They are expensive, unnecessary additions to a good diet and teach our kids nothing about good food, or even what good food should taste like. Our children will get all the nutrients they need to thrive from naturally low-calorie foodstuffs, such as meat, eggs, fish, yoghurts, fruit and vegetables as well as lots more.

In the following chapters the plan will emerge that will give your children all the nutrients and variety they require, while keeping excess calories at bay, therefore helping to keep their weight at an appropriate level.

Rule 6:

Say 'No' to passive consumption

We need our children to eat and enjoy good food. We want them to look at it, taste it, thoroughly relish it, finish what they want to eat of it and leave the table. What we do not want is our children consuming hundreds of calories in excess of their requirement, every day, without even noticing them going down. Extra calories often go past their lips in the form of drinks and snack foods. Today's trend towards smoothies, juices, sports drinks, breakfast bars and snacking in general is giving our kids a constant urge to eat, as they see others doing. *This needs to stop.* It needs to stop today. Not only is constant grazing throughout the day adding endless extra calories to their intake, it is also causing them to lose interest in good-quality, plain foods. When their tastebuds become accustomed to foods that always taste sweet or salty, as snack foods tend to, they rarely want to eat anything but food that is overly sweetened and overly salted, so the notion of a Brussels sprout for dinner can horrify because of its relative blandness.

Truth be told, our kids are getting very little value or satisfaction from this way of eating. They are rarely allowed to be hungry any more; it is almost an imprisonable offence to allow it. Yet our kids will eat at dinner time, having already squeezed in a calorie-laden snack since lunch. This may have been called an afternoon snack, but I call it a disaster waiting to happen. If they consume too many calories at snack time they will lose interest in vegetables and simple foods when they are not adequately hungry at mealtime. This is a problem. **The consumption of unnecessary calories is the primary reason for weight gain.** There is no mystery to this. Excessive snacking may, in fact, be at the heart of the problem that is our kids' habits around food today. Excess calories being taken in on a consistent basis leads to fat being stored in cells: this is very simple science.

About fifteen years ago, while travelling, I was in Fiji, where many of the tourists are Australian. In one particular resort I can recall seeing some overweight Australian children pottering by the pool with their families. It really surprised me to see Australian children who were so overweight. We all know how outdoors a way of life people live in Australia, as do the Kiwis we knew when we lived in New Zealand. It took me a couple of days to notice the coloured wristbands these kids were wearing and what the colours meant. They were members of a very exclusive club, of which I, being at the time young, recently married and free of kids, knew nothing. They were 'all-in' or 'full-board' customers. This 'all-in' approach meant that the kids could present themselves at the pool-side bar at any hour of the day or night and get a container full of their favourite soft drink. They were also entitled to any amount of ice cream they wanted. They did not require sign-off from parents: in fact they did not appear to need any sort of permission at all. It was literally an 'all you can eat' approach to treat foods for them for the duration of their week's holiday.

To put this in terms of calories, if you were to allow your child a very reasonable-looking 250ml bottle of fizzy drink every day for a week, and accompany that with just one bar of milk chocolate (as you might on a wet week's holiday in Ireland) you would be providing them with 500kcals in excess of their meals for the seven days of your holiday. This would add up to a staggering 3,500kcals. As you now know, this would have gained them a pound of fat in that week, unless you took them off for a two-hour jaunt up a mountain every one of those days to help work off the excess calories. Can you imagine the calorie damage a child can do when left to their own devices for a week or two?

Sadly, fifteen years on, these 'all-in' packages have become quite commonplace in family-centred holiday resorts. We are being encouraged to buy off our kids by feeding them ad infinitum, which of course leaves us to get a little more rest and freedom on what is our holiday too. Don't get me wrong, I am a great believer in bribery when it comes to kids. I think bribery is the way forward. The currency should not be food, though; instead, let it be the freedom to explore the resort or to stay up late and watch the show with the adults, or perhaps allowing them that trinket they had their eye on in some vending machine. Don't let it be fizzy drinks and ice cream and sweets. It is our responsibility, as adults, to keep them from such harm.

Another example of passive consumption is going to the cinema, which is often considered 'family time', say on a Saturday, after a hard week of homework and activities. This 'treat' for the kids can soar beyond all reason in terms of calorie intake. Go to the cinema as entertainment in its own right by all means. But separate it from the act of eating. If you go for an ice cream after the cinema, then great. This is most certainly the stuff of treats. What we tend to do, however, is quite different. We might buy a bagful of sweets, plus a drink for the kids, plus, possibly, the box of popcorn that you could almost sit into and eat your way out of! This is too much entirely. From a calorie perspective, it can mount up into the many hundreds, possibly well over a thousand, calories per person. For one snack. This is not helping our kids to achieve balance: this is hindering their efforts. The real problem here is that our kids will consume this calorific bombshell passively. They will hardly register it. They will be too busy watching the movie to notice exactly how much they are eating. More damaging, in the long term, is the fact that they will always associate watching a movie with eating. This habit may well stick for life. Before you know it the 'goodies' even come out while watching the television at home in the evening. I see this trend all the time when dealing with adults who want to lose weight. One of the greatest challenges for many to deal with is this need to snack at night while watching television. This is one habit you do not want to pass on to your kids. Separate the two activities. Go for food *after* the movie – if it is time to eat, that is.

Going to the cinema is often considered 'family time', say on a Saturday, after a hard week of homework and activities. This 'treat' for the kids can soar beyond all reason in terms of calorie intake. Go to the cinema as entertainment in its own right by all means. Separate it from the act of eating.

For some of us, this is already part and parcel of the day's entertainment: we already have strong associations between food and film watching. If my approach seems too big a step to take straight off the bat, then damage limitation should be your initial aim.

When you go to the cinema, bring with you, from home or the local shop, a small bag of popcorn, for instance, or a regular packet of sweets for each child. Allow them a much more reasonable amount than they would buy if left to their own devices at the sweet stand at the cinema. Not only will you save calories but you will also save a lot of money, as prices in the cinema tend to be outrageously high.

Portion control has to be central to the consumption of such high-calorie treats. If you leave the decision on what constitutes a portion to the cinema staff, you are putting it in the wrong hands. We need to take total control here. The kids can either have a small treat at the cinema or they can wait until after the cinema to get a bigger one. The lure of a snack after the cinema instead of a 'small' treat at the cinema might tempt them to dispense with the movie snack altogether, in time. Perhaps they will go to the cinema with nothing and build up an appetite for their Sunday treat after the movie. You may wish to take this staggered approach to ease the transition to snack-free movies. I can acknowledge that this approach is not a quick fix, but it does work and it is certainly worth the effort.

Only recently, I had the joy of going to a children's concert with my three older children, while my husband stayed at home with the smallest one. I went, with tickets in hand, looking forward to the fun – which we had. What I genuinely forgot about (not usually being the one to bring them to such events) was the array of offerings available for consumption during the extended mid-way break. Two boys next to us turned up with very large blue 'slushies' and a large box of popcorn each. Others around us ate ice creams and sweets. My poor left-out kids! What amazed me was how many fat kids there were in the audience. This was, in fact, an energetic concert designed to get kids dancing in the aisles and the irony was not lost on me when I looked around during the second half of the concert to see that most kids were more stationary than before because they were busy consuming their sweets. Mine danced their hearts out and, incidentally, went home at eight to a lovely (pre-planned) hot chocolate and cookie treat.

'Pizza night' in front of our favourite Saturday night television programme is now also considered 'normal'. The 'experts' (in marketing) have deemed it to be a very ordinary part of a family night in. I would argue strongly against this trend. If passively watching television while passively consuming hundreds upon hundreds of calories is considered the norm, it is not an appropriate one. Eat dinner at dinner time. Sit down with the kids to watch your favourite programme later. **Do not eat while watching television.**

Saturday evening television is full of food ads. Is this a coincidence? No. It is because the food companies hope to get you and your kids to eat more. Did you know that many of the major global food corporations have marketing divisions dedicated to creating brand loyalty in their customers from the age of two? We, as parents, need to be aware of this fact and aim to immunise our kids against such aggressive advertising campaigns. By definition, advertising creates a need where there wasn't one before. And it works. Within a very few years, what would have been considered a rare and, in fact, unexpected treat – a takeaway pizza at eight o'clock on a Saturday evening – has recently become utterly acceptable. How did this happen so fast? It is quite a coup on the part of the takeaway providers: we needed little or no convincing that this is acceptable behaviour. I am constantly amazed by how many families embrace this very new way of eating.

The marketing 'gurus' saw a gap in the market that highlights to us hard-working parents that we might need a night off from cooking and that we also want to sit down for 'family time' in front of the television. We deserve the break. We can spend this 'quality' time together. Put a great big pizza with all the trimmings and extras into the mix and we have a recipe for success. What could possibly be wrong with this picture? What might be *very* wrong with this picture is that in this scenario our kids are eating very late; they are eating passively; and they are consuming too many calories from fat and too much salt. As often as not, they are consuming bucketloads of sugar in the form of drinks or ice cream to boot. They are learning, from your example, that eating while watching television is appropriate. Of course, the fizzy drink consumed with the meal contains far too much sugar for a child at this time of night (or, indeed at any time, if too many of these drinks are allowed). Their system is exposed to so much sugar that they get a late-night 'high' (no going to bed early that night!) followed by a very cranky 'low'.

You will have seen this described somewhere over the years but I think it's worth illustrating the effect here. One of the biggest health issues American children, for instance, face at the moment is that of type 2 diabetes, also called adult-onset diabetes. Consistently exposing your child's system to too much sugar (more than 85g a day), by allowing them to constantly snack on sugary foods – including such foods as sugar-coated breakfast cereals, flavoured milks and sodas – their insulin-producing system (the pancreas) is being over-worked and can become exhausted. This is occurring more and more at the moment and this is how it looks in the blood.

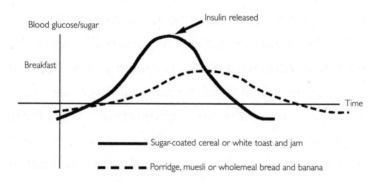

You can see from the illustration that when a high-sugar, low-fibre breakfast is eaten, there is a sudden release of sugar into the blood (a sugar 'high'). It is the job of the pancreas to release insulin at this point, to bring sugar out of the blood and into the cells, as otherwise it would prove dangerous to health. By comparison, when a high-fibre breakfast is eaten, it takes time to release the sugar from the fibre matrix, through chewing and digesting the oats or wholewheat bread, say. Blood sugar therefore rises more slowly and does not give the 'high' that comes from the sugary cereal: and as a result, less insulin is released to bring the blood-sugar level down slowly.

If we allow our kids to eat mainly the high-sugar, refined version of foods (sugar-, honey- or cocoa-coated cereals, biscuits, smoothies, breakfast bars, flavoured milks, ice creams) they run the risk of not only gaining unnecessary fat but of also exhausting this otherwise accurate insulin feedback mechanism, which for the most part works perfectly well.

While in the long term a potentially exhausted insulin-producing system is putting our kids at serious risk of ill health and a shorter life span, especially if there is diabetes in the family, in the more immediate term you end up with a cranky child on a sugar 'low' and in a rotten mood, through no fault of their own!

More recently we have been subjected to variations on the pizza theme. The inventor of the liquid cheese crust in pizzas should have been certified insane, in my opinion. It is now deemed acceptable that we add as many poor-quality saturated fats to our foods as physically possible. As a result of this genius, we can now order a pizza with a cheese-filled crust for our delectation. Heaven forbid our crust should be plain and boring. Do we need to utilise every single opportunity to maximise the calorie intake of our family? I think not. Recently, a double decker pizza made its way onto takeaway menus. Another moment of genius! This is another poor trend, directing us in precisely the wrong direction, away from a moderate, healthy approach to food. We do not need to maximise every opportunity to get calories into our kids: we need neither to fill our pizza crusts with cheese nor double the load per bite.

Have you noticed how the pizza deals are often designed so that it is nearly impossible not to be tempted into also buying the two-litre bottle of fizzy drink, the garlic bread and the ice cream to accompany your pizza? This is marketing a concept aimed at you – the bargain 'meal deal'. Resist. Have pizza for dinner by all means. A pizza or two in your freezer is a great stand-by. Spend the same fifteen minutes it would take to get your takeaway pizza setting the table for dinner, assembling a salad and perhaps organising dessert. Sit down (say at seven p.m.) to a couple of slices of pizza per person with your family and perhaps a glass of wine for you, the hard-working parent. Accompany it with the family's favourite salad ingredients, either assembled to taste or arranged as single ingredients in containers on the table. Have a little ice cream with strawberries for dessert. Then watch television. Eat, clear up, then turn on the television and relax.

Separate the two activities. You deserve it. They deserve it.

There is little better than the smell of a roast dinner cooking in the oven. Christmas dinner comes to mind when I think of the ultimate roast, when the turkey is in the oven for so long that the entire house starts to smell of turkey, stuffing and, of course, roast potatoes. It is so tantalising that you salivate in anticipation of it all morning and it is hard to wait until lunchtime to eat it. You would love to be able to sneak a few morsels without anyone noticing, but you cannot. The appetite you build up in this scenario, to me, represents how we should feel before every meal, every day of the year, with no exception.

If you have ever woken up 'starving' you will remember how good the plainest of porridge would have tasted that morning. You would have been drawn to a substantial bowl of something wholesome, like porridge or muesli, not necessarily the sugary cereal you might love on a not-so-hungry morning. Having eaten this substantial bowl of cereal you would have felt full and content and gone happily about your business. If you were to wake up not so hungry, you would feel more like picking at morsels of food for the day. Before you know it, you are having coffee and a Danish pastry at eleven, to fix your desire for sugar, not to relieve hunger. This is clearly not ideal.

Eating purely for the sake of enjoyment is a recipe for weight gain. We really need to work on this notion of listening to our appetite and paying close attention to feelings of hunger and satiety (fullness). If we can do this ourselves, then we can teach our kids next. So practise this yourself first. Stop eating late at night so that you get to wake up hungrier than you are used to in the morning. I often get weight-loss clients to chew gum for the first three or four nights, to underline this point. We often eat at ten and eleven at night, when we are peckish, not hungry, because we saw a food ad on the television, or because we know there is left-over cheesecake in the fridge, or simply because we have multi-packs of treats in the house that we can dive into on the merest whim.

Perhaps alcohol is making us feel hungry. Ironically, we love to have savoury snacks with a glass of wine or beer at night, though we are already consuming calories in the beverage itself. It might shock you to realise that the 200g packet of roasted peanuts you might share at night with your loved one contains a staggering 1,200kcal. This is a day's eating for someone on a weight-reducing diet. The wine, per generous glass (is there any other type?) comes in at about 180kcal. Share a bottle between two and you have consumed a further 300kcals. If, as an experiment, you spent tonight, tomorrow night and the night after *not eating* past dinner time you would begin to wake up good and hungry every morning. In about three short days you would bounce out of bed in the mornings, hungrily looking forward to your bowl of shredded wheat, spelt puffs or oats. Suddenly you are on track to listening more closely to your natural appetite. This, incidentally, feels wonderful.

When you listen to your signals of hunger you are in a position to listen to your signals of feeling full. Leave the table at eighty per cent full and by lunchtime you will be very keen to have a hearty and wholesome meal. You would not spoil the promise and enjoyment of your planned lunch by eating a Danish pastry at eleven, just because someone put it in your path. This is how we need to teach our kids to start trusting their feelings of 'hunger' and 'fullness' again. We are equipped with these skills when we are young. Have you ever noticed how a three-year-old can leave some chocolate or ice cream on their plate after dinner? We would be virtually incapable of leaving chocolate behind us, as, incidentally, would an eight-year-old. Somewhere between the ages of about three and six we learn how to enjoy food for its own sake rather than for its simple function as fuel. In other words, unless the urge to eat ice cream purely for its sweetness and unctuousness was tempered by household rules about not eating too much of it, we would have eaten ice cream in preference to dinner any day we got away with it. Yes, I exaggerate here, but not as wildly as you might think. If you pay attention to the picky kids in your sphere you will notice that, while they may not eat your lovingly prepared shepherd's pie for dinner, they will rarely say 'No' to the dessert that follows it. They may not eat the breakfast you prepared for them, but give them a bowl of frosted flakes and watch what happens. So we do, indeed, in many cases allow our kids to give in to their preference for sweet and high-fat foods. We simply might not be aware of this fact.

Many cereals, for instance, that are labelled 'healthy' contain far too much added sugar to be wholesome. When food is shaped in an unnatural way it is a highly processed food. Yes, there might be whole grains in there somewhere, but so too is a large quantity of sugar and salt. Just because a cereal is fortified with vitamins and minerals it is not necessarily wholesome. We love the notion of providing our kids with a nutritional insurance policy in the name of fortification. This is the same reason we buy chewy sweet-like vitamin and mineral supplements for our kids in winter to ward off colds and flu. Having worked in the supplement industry, let me just say that no pill can ever replace the myriad nutritional benefits of whole food: foods you can name. We owe it to our kids to think about this. We owe our kids not to give in to their desire for processed and sweet foods only, even when these are marketed as good food. We need to insist that they eat breakfast, lunch and dinner as stand-alone meals. They do not need to clear their plates at every sitting. Dessert or treats come after the main meal, as long as some of everything on the plate has at least been tried.

Passive consumption, as represented by the example of the Danish pastry, needs to be avoided at all costs by our kids, if we want them to maintain a healthy weight. Rule number five, from today, has to be to **SAY 'NO' TO PASSIVE CONSUMPTION.**

The consumption of what are marketed as 'healthy choices' is also proving problematic to our children, in my opinion. Smoothies (liquidised fruits and fruit juices) represent a current trend towards passive consumption in our children's food habits. The theory, used by those marketing them to us, is that if your child drinks them down in one go you can guarantee that they will get at least part of their recommended daily intake of fruit and vegetables. Great. Nutrition in a bottle. Life is easy as a result of these wonder drinks.

I do not agree. If your child were sick or recovering from an illness, a smoothie might be a useful tool in your repertoire for getting your child to take in some nourishment, when their appetite is not what it should be. When your child is fit and well, however, I have to disagree with their marketing of these products.

Our kids have a built-in ability to chew food (they have a mouthful of teeth and strong jaw muscles) and by doing so they register in their brain that this mechanical action is going on. When you eat an apple in its entirety, your brain knows that seventy or so calories were consumed in the effort that was involved in biting, chewing and swallowing it and in most instances one apple will suffice. Our kids do not generally ask for a second one.

In contrast, with a smoothie an equivalent number of calories is very often gone in the first swig out of the bottle. A child can comfortably consume the entire contents, at a possible 250kcals, without feeling in the least full. Why? Because they do not spend a moment chewing and chomping their way through those calories; they can let them slide very easily down their throat with very little effort involved. The same can be said for chocolate, banana or strawberry milk. You know I am a great fan of dairy products, but not when doctored with enormous amounts of added sugar and flavourings. Spot the difference? I call that passive consumption. Even though the child is taking in milk products or (sometimes, not always) good-quality fruit, they are making none of the conscious effort we are hoping to get them to put into their eating.

When consuming that number of calories I strongly believe our kids should be able to see them on the plate, for example the six grapes, half an apple, ten raspberries, half a banana, twenty blueberries and pot of yoghurt the drink would have promised to deliver.

Believe it or not, that amount of calories equates to one adult-sized bar of chocolate, yet because it comes under the heading of fruit we believe that children entirely benefit from it. Again, to achieve 250kcal from fruit your child could have consumed quite a plateful, over the course of the day, at appropriate snack times, and avoided the need for any such drink.

Initially, you may find it difficult to shift your approach from passively eating to consciously sitting down to eat, even at snack time, if it is not what you currently do as a family. Trust me: promising the kids ice cream after the cinema, when the entire family sits down to eat it, in an ice cream parlour, will win them over very quickly. Eating good fruit they enjoy will prove no hardship. Essentially, calling a spade a spade will serve them very well in the long run. When they want to eat fruit, that is what they should get. Then, when it is time (on occasion) to have chocolate, that is what they get. I see no role for the breakfast cereal bar that is laden with more sugar than you can shake a stick at, that pretends to be wholesome food and is consumed regularly by kids safe in the knowledge that their parents are happy to feed it to them. There would, in most cases, be less sugar in a little chocolate bar.

Remember, Rome wasn't built in a day. They will initially argue about not getting sweets for the movie, or complain that they do not have cereal bars in their lunchboxes any more, but when they see how the new trend works out – in their favour – they will soon give in. Be brave. Stick to your guns. It is a lesson worth passing on to your kids. Separate eating from other activities. The rewards are good habits around food, for life. They may thank you some day.

Rule 7:
Eat only when you feel hungry

Our children need in the region of fourteen to eighteen hundred calories per day from food. I have no intention of breaking foods down into calories and nutrient content. This information is available in any library book on nutrition and hardly makes for scintillating reading! In this context it would provide too much information, it could prove too distracting and, at any rate, no child should ever be on a calorie-restricted diet, in my opinion. While we adults might have become preoccupied with the calorie, carbohydrate and fat content of foods, we should do our kids the favour of not involving them in this near-obsessive behaviour. I hate the idea of children discussing the fact that chocolate is fattening or that sweets are bad for you. They should not concern themselves with any such misinformed notions. Kids should never know about calories, in terms of food restriction.

Dieting does not work. If it did, you would follow one corrective 'diet' phase in your life, if and when necessary, and that would be an end to it. This is rarely, if ever, the case. Kids need to avoid the apparently almost inevitable 'dieting' future we are leading them towards. They should know, instead, that chocolate is good for them, if and when they are hungry for it, and if they have eaten their balanced meal beforehand. Kids also need to enjoy sweets, any sweets, as fun food, with no guilt involved and no idea that they are not beneficial to health. **Food should be fun for kids.** When your kids have eaten their fruit, yoghurt and sandwich for lunch in school and have had, say, swimming lessons that afternoon, they can be so ravenously hungry on the way home that there is no reason not to allow them some sweets, as a fun treat. They appreciate the gesture and there is no harm in a little of what they fancy, on occasion. It will do them good. It will do you good to see your children having a healthy relationship with sweets and treats as well as with wholesome food. Balance is what we are hoping to achieve, overall.

We tend, as adults, to restrict our consumption of certain foods and allow ourselves to eat only particular foods that adhere to the set of rules we have set up for ourselves in our mind. Perhaps you only eat 'diet' yoghurts or consume only wholemeal crackers, or would never allow yourself to eat a banana or a grape, on the assumption that they are fattening. These rules, often based on shaky, inaccurate scientific grounds, will have come about as a reaction to what you feel keeps you on the straight and narrow, weight-wise.

Whether these rules work for you is another story. Sometimes they may work, but in other cases they do not, as having stringent rules about food can very often lead to 'binge' eating. We are all familiar with this notion of restricting something so much that when we eventually have some of it we want more and more, until we eat too much of it. When this happens, we feel like a failure, which of course puts the weight issue back on the agenda, out come the rules again and we aim to adhere to them even more stringently this time. This keeps our habits in order until we succumb to the next temptation, and so it goes. If we do not allow ourselves to eat foods that are high in fat or high in carbohydrate content and end up eating crackers for lunch with spreadable cheese or, heaven forbid, such delicacies as sugar-free jelly, we are most certainly missing out on a myriad of nutrients that these foods will not supply.

Why do we adhere to such restrictive eating? The answer might be that we have run out of ideas in our quest for the perfect diet. Because we might have exhausted all avenues of trying to restrict ourselves around our favourite foods, we fall prey to the marketing of so-called 'diet' foods which, when consumed as meals, leave us hungry, undernourished and miserable. We feel 'safe' and 'controlled' under the influence of the marketing of these diet foods when that is all we consume. If I could assure you here and now that you need never again purchase or consume a sad and sorry 'diet' food and you will not gain weight, I think you would be pretty happy. I can and I will.

If you eat only when you are hungry, you can eat whatever you wish, within reason, and never put on unnecessary weight. The 'within reason' part of the argument means that you do have to follow a balanced approach to meals, as illustrated by the lunch/dinner plate idea discussed on page 161. At the end of the meal, if you feel full (ideally only eighty per cent full), you will not consume the chocolate bar with your name on it that you squirreled away! However, if you find yourself wanting, perhaps, only one slice of bread with your salad and meat for lunch instead of your usual two slices, thus 'leaving room' for the chocolate bar, then you should sit down with a cup of tea and enjoy it. Make it a small bar, one you actually want, not one you think you 'should' have. In calorie terms this small bar equates roughly to one buttered slice of bread. When 'allowed' you will be less likely to overdo it and binge on the rest of the multi-pack (which, by the way, is no longer in your cupboard).

Chicken or Fish with Red Pesto

We might be under the impression that because we need to keep our foods 'low fat' at all times that we have to eat our chicken either steamed or baked dry. This makes for miserable eating and, as we all know, the cure for feeling constantly miserable is to eat chocolate, much chocolate! The same goes for our kids: we need to feed them tasty food, not fat-free fare. Thus was born my instant tasty chicken recipe that uses only two ingredients: chicken (or fish) and pesto, bought from the supermarket.

Ingredients

✓ I chicken breast per adult/half a breast per small child, or I small piece of haddock/cod per small child and 2 pieces per adult

✓ I heaped teaspoon red pesto or sun-dried tomato paste

Method

• Place the chicken or fish on tinfoil or a baking tray and spread the pesto on top. Cook in an oven at 180°C for 25 minutes (for the chicken) or 20 minutes (for the fish).

• Serve with plenty of green vegetables and perhaps home-made potato wedges (see page 94) or magic mash (next recipe). This is one of my all-time stand-by dinners. It is foolproof and on the table within thirty minutes. When I seem to have nothing fresh in the house I will always have frozen white fish and frozen green vegetables and, of course, a plentiful supply of potatoes is always in residence. The dish works best, in fact, when the fish is frozen.

Magic Mash

I remember serving this with dinner to my sister's husband, along with the horde. He remarked that it was so nice that there must be cream in it. Let me assure you there is not!

Ingredients

✓ To serve four, you will need approximately five medium-sized potatoes (the kids will eat a smaller portion than the adults)

✓ a pinch of salt and pepper

✓ 1 teaspoon of dried thyme

✓ approx. 1 cup low-fat milk

Method

• Peel the potatoes and boil, steam or microwave until they are soft and fluffy.

• Next, add the salt, pepper and herbs and mash well with the potatoes.

• Then add the milk and continue to mash until the potatoes become creamy and sloppy. The 'yummy' factor comes from this 'creaminess'!

꿍꿍

Dieting has become a way of life for many of us. We eat 'low-fat' and 'diet' biscuit bars, an oxymoron if ever there was one, in the name of healthy eating. We should feel at ease having an occasional biscuit bar: the full-fat version that satisfies our need for fat and sugar in that moment. Our kids should not grow up under the grim impression that all adults ever get as treats are these insipid, unsatisfying poor relations to the real thing. Instead of passing on this unhealthy 'dieting' way of life to our kids, my aim in writing this book is to equip you with the tools – and a few tricks – to get your child to eat a balanced diet, full of nutrients and full of enjoyment. Then they also get to eat real treats on occasion. This is normal eating. This is how we used to eat as children (if you are over thirty years of age at any rate).

When you try it out for yourself you will realise how liberating is this idea of eating only when you are hungry. Your child, who once knew this trick – until perhaps the age of three or four – can learn it again and will stop nagging you for treats once they feel satisfied. Your child's diet can be moderate in calories, while never including anything they 'hate' to eat. **I also want you to constantly work on broadening their food horizons.** Of course, they will say 'No' more often than not to anything new, as you know, but time will take care of that particular issue. You know that when a child is hungry they will be more willing to try a new food. Therefore, the work you will have done on stamping out passive consumption of foods will have created this hunger we are looking for at each and every mealtime.

Cat-food Tagine

My kids christened this one! It is, in fact, lamb tagine that comes out of the oven so dark that, to the kids, it resembles what the cat eats – only in looks, let me assure you, not in taste! This tagine takes an hour and a half in the oven, so it is not a quick-fix dinner. It does, however, take very little effort on your part and can be eaten a few days after it was first made. I often make double quantities and serve it again later in the week, when it tastes almost better than it did on first cooking. As the basis of a leftovers dinner it really does work well. Kids will only eat a small amount of this, as it is dense, but also sweet, so I serve it with lots of greens and either couscous or mashed potatoes.

Ingredients

✓ 1 large onion, peeled and chopped

✓ 2 tablespoons olive oil

✓ approx. 400g diced leg or neck of lamb

✓ spices (most of which are probably sitting in your cupboards right now, gathering dust): ½ teaspoon cinnamon; ½ teaspoon turmeric; ½ teaspoon ground ginger; ½ teaspoon cumin; ½ teaspoon allspice

✓ 500ml water

✓ a few dates (perhaps 6–8) without stones, chopped into small pieces

✓ a good pinch of salt

Method

- Brown the onion in the oil in a heavy-bottomed casserole dish on the cooker top. Add the lamb and brown for two to three minutes. Add all the spices and stir around for another two to three minutes. Then add the water, chopped dates and salt and place in the oven at approximately 150°C (or leave on a low heat on the hob) for one and a half hours. When it comes out the lamb is meltingly tender and sweet.

≈

The most basic rule of thumb, also rule number seven, is **EAT ONLY WHEN YOU FEEL HUNGRY.** If this rule were adhered to, we would not have overweight children. If your kids could spot feelings of hunger, they could spot the feeling of being full. If they are eating before they even register hunger, they are, by definition, overeating. Think about it. As you might teach your child to look right and left before crossing the road, so too you can teach them to spot how their appetite works. I find that one of my own children, for instance, at six years of age, still needs to be taught this. While my two eldest can happily leave food on the plate behind them, and go on to ask for dessert, my six-year-old has not yet fine-tuned her sense of feeling full so as to be able to resist finishing her favourite dinner (which happens to be roast chicken). She will go on to eat dessert until she feels 'stuffed', as she might eloquently put it. Unless I ask her, towards the end of dinner, 'Have you had enough? Do you want to leave some room for dessert?' she will clear her plate. If I do not intervene, she will, even at the age of six, quite often overeat: in the short term she will feel the worse for wear; and in the long term possibly end up with a weight problem.

Children up to the age of three or four, for the most part, know instinctively when they are full. A very young child can usually leave lots on the plate behind them, even sweet foods, if they are full. An older child, by age five or six certainly, has developed the ability to over-ride feelings of being full and will quite often go on to enjoy more sweet things, just because they like them, not because they are hungry. In my house I ask them to eat some of everything on the plate at dinner time. They do not need to clear their plate unless they are hungry enough to do so. Leaving room for dessert means that they get used to the idea of finishing before they are completely full, and this in itself is a very valuable lesson to impart.

As I mentioned earlier in this book, the Japanese have a saying that we should leave the table at eighty per cent full. This sounds like a life of misery! It is not. What it achieves is a wealth of energy after eating that we often miss out on. If you think of the most exaggerated case, which in my world would be represented by Christmas day, of eating to 'beyond full', you will be able to acknowledge that we are fit for nothing after dinner but snoring at the ceiling, with the top button on our waistband opened. The opposite scenario is to leave the table at a level of fullness that would be eight on a scale of one to ten. Twenty minutes later, you feel full. It can, in fact, take up to forty minutes to feel completely full. The difference is that you feel full and energised, not weighed down by your last meal. And so it is for our kids.

> A very young child can usually leave lots on the plate behind them, even sweet foods, if they are full. An older child, by age five or six certainly, has developed the ability to over-ride feelings of being full and will quite often go on to enjoy more sweet things, just because they like them, not because they are hungry.

The principles that I adhere to are, therefore, that children eat only when they are hungry and that they finish before they are too full. This means that some days they might not want an afternoon snack, for instance, but the payback is that they are very hungry for dinner and eat plenty of the good stuff. Cereals, breads and starchy vegetables should form the basis of your child's three meals a day. Carbohydrates are the fuel in our kids' engine. For breakfast they can have wholemeal cereals – or refined cereals, within reason, as long as they are not sugary. Some examples are porridge or muesli with low-fat milk (as recommended by health professionals for everyone over the age of two) and a banana, or two wheat biscuits with blueberries on top and milk, or bran flakes and a yoghurt. Or wholemeal toast with butter and marmalade and a glass of milk, or a plain bagel with peanut butter and jam with a plum or a pot of yoghurt.

If your child had a good breakfast, which they ate sitting down, they will want no more than a light mid-morning snack. As you know by now, this will constitute a piece of fruit only. If they are hungrier, a piece of fruit and a little pot of yoghurt or chunk of cheese would be suitable. If you structure breakfast around a carbohydrate (starchy food), you will find it easy to get a milk-based product (yoghurt, milk or cheese) and fruit portion in there to accompany it.

Similarly, lunch gets constructed around the chosen carbohydrate. Let's say the sandwich reigns. It certainly does in my house. Whether your child has ham, cheese, tuna, chicken, peanut butter, eggs or something else is up to them and you to decide. What is important is that the sandwich contains a portion of protein-rich foods, such as those I have listed. The rule of being able to name every ingredient off the top of your head applies very much here. In other words, processed meats, slices of meat with a face stamped on them, or rubbery looking meat-like products should never get a look-in. Where, for instance, does a 'turkey rasher' come from on the body of a turkey? Keep it real. This is also a good opportunity to get in another 'milk' hit: cheese in a sandwich. We are looking for up to five portions of milk products per day as the child goes from toddler to teen. Alternatively, drinking milk is one very good habit to get your child into at this stage.

What goes with the sandwich? Clearly we need a vegetable 'hit'. Otherwise we have little hope of achieving our four portions today. Cucumber sticks, baby tomatoes, lettuce in a sandwich, vegetable soup in a flask, celery sticks all come to mind. Your children will surprise you when it comes to what they like to crunch on. If your child is going through a growth spurt, and always hungry, you could add another piece of fruit. In the worst-case scenario they will bring it home on days they didn't need it. Any left-over lunchtime fruit turns into the first part of their after-school snack in my house. While I realise this sounds a little mean, my aim is to get that next fruit snack included as soon as they are hungry again. You will immediately notice that they are good and hungry for dinner later when their afternoon snack was nothing more than a piece of fruit. Fruit and a cereal with milk for an after-school snack on a hungry day works very well, I find.

Dummy's Brown Bread

No insult intended! The dummy here refers to me and the fact that I can whip up this fabulously tasty and ferociously nutritious bread in a matter of seconds. Kids love it and it has seeds in it; in most bread these are two mutually exclusive features.

Ingredients

✓ 150g wholemeal flour

✓ 200g white flour

✓ 1 teaspoon bread soda

✓ ¼ teaspoon salt

✓ 2 tablespoons mixed seeds, e.g. linseeds, sunflower seeds, pumpkin seeds

✓ 600ml buttermilk

Method

• Mix all the dry ingredients together in a large bowl. Add the buttermilk and stir gently together. Pour into a 2lb non-stick loaf tin that has been sprayed with spray oil and place in a preheated oven at 160°C for 50–60 minutes.

I look on plain cereals, even cornflakes, as a very convenient vehicle for milk. Our kids do not need high-fibre foods at all times since they can find too much fibre a little more abrasive than adults do and can end up with sudden urges to go to the loo. Also, if you switch them to a very high-fibre diet they can miss out on some valuable nutrients by not having the appetite to consume other foods because they are feeling so full from the fibre. A slice of toast with what we call 'banana jam' (the most squashed uneaten lunchbox banana) is a favourite afternoon snack with my kids.

Dinner will be thoroughly enjoyed by the whole family when we can all sit down, hungry, to a dinner that we love. My husband fought this idea for a number of years. As we went through what seemed to him endless years of high chairs and tantrums at the table, he favoured the idea of feeding the kids first and then us sitting down to our dinner later, like civilised people! Of course, this is what I wanted too, so we did this for quite a few years. You know the scenario of having to feed kids on their schedule with bland, mushy dinners you wouldn't touch with a ten-foot bargepole yourself? Of course you do. One of my own favourite Friday treats, after a long week's work, was plonking my two-year-old in front of the television with me while I ate my Chinese takeaway. My husband would be working late, and I was heavily pregnant with my second child. I felt, at the time, that I could just about justify this behaviour, as my daughter would have eaten at the child-minder's house earlier and I would be exhausted after a hard week. And, of course, she would never remember. I'm glad to say this worked out, but only just. In the few short years it took for my kids to get to the age when they question me about everything and will certainly remember everything, I realised that the evening meal, at the very least, should be eaten 'en famille', every evening, with no exceptions.

If I thought I could eat my (different) dinner in front of the television and expect them to happily eat theirs at the table, I would be sadly mistaken. Monkey see, monkey do. The day would come when one of them would expect to be allowed to eat their dinner on the sofa too. So this is a discipline for me to adhere to: the 'eat only at the table' rule. Let me reassure you, though, that it really pays off. Sitting and having dinner with the horde is one of the highlights of my day now; and even my husband loves it. One of the kids always gets the job of setting the table, another is waiter or waitress. The only question I am ever asked is 'Am I setting it for five or for six?', as one of them might be eating at a friend's house.

So what should dinner look like? The same as lunch, in structure. If I were to draw it for you, your plate would be a circle, with half the circle containing only vegetables (salad, soup, fresh or frozen); one quarter containing 'meat' (meat, eggs, cheese or fish); and the final quarter containing carbohydrate (rice, beans, corn, potatoes or pasta). Fat would form a little circle in the middle of the plate (oil, butter, cream, crème fraîche).

Some examples might be: lasagne and salad (not chips – the carbohydrate is accounted for in the pasta); fish fingers, beans, peas and broccoli (the beans count as the carbohydrate); chicken, potatoes, carrots and sugar snaps; salmon with oven chips (ideally home-made) with sweetcorn and green beans and the obligatory ketchup; scrambled egg with toast and tomatoes (eggs count for the protein in this meal); chickpea curry (or chicken and chickpea curry), incorporating peas and cauliflower, with rice. You get the idea. If this structure is adhered to, the kids can eat their favourite dinners every day. The structure achieves balance; and **balance is what we want, not dieting, restriction, hunger, hardship.** Remember, kids need fat in every meal, so we do not necessarily need to go down the steamed white fish route; we can fry our white fish in olive oil. Let them enjoy their favourites, as long as they eat some of everything on the plate.

When consulting with clients I represent the dinner and lunch plate like this:

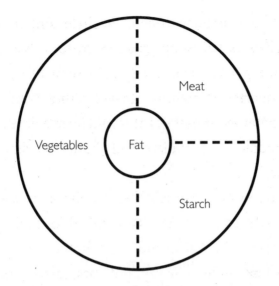

The ease of visualising your child's plate (as well as your own) like this allows you to take all the guesswork out of the process of feeding them. So does pizza represent a balanced meal? Yes, if it is accompanied by a side salad or salad components. Does pizza with garlic bread and ice cream represent a balanced meal? No. It is far too high in refined carbohydrates, sugar, salt and fat.

We often have dessert in my house; in fact we have it every day. I have nothing against dessert. I favour it greatly and it works wonders. I mentioned in Rule 3 that weekday dessert consists of fruit and 'milk', such as stewed apple and custard or pears and yoghurt. At the weekend, it gets upgraded to the likes of apple crumble and ice cream or pear and chocolate sponge with custard. Remember, food is there to be relished. Enjoy food with your kids. This is how they learn to enjoy good food themselves. Give them foods that they enjoy eating, but with the formality that may currently be lacking. Over time, often a lengthy period of time, they will develop a sense of enthusiasm for and interest in good food again, in all its variety of tastes, colours and textures, and any weight issue will resolve itself.

There is another side to weight management in kids that cannot be overlooked. It is energy expenditure. We need to get our kids to expend more calories every day. How do we get our kids to use more energy than they consume (which currently they tend not to)? Next I will break down this necessary energy expenditure into two parts. Achieving it is simpler than you might think. It does not have to cost a cent to maintain and kids enjoy doing it. Trust me, you will benefit too.

Rule 8:

Get moving!

Movement and exercise are two different things. We commonly get these mixed up, thinking that they are one and the same. Movement really relates to a state of mind. We tend to be either 'movers' or 'non-movers' in my experience of dealing with people. Exercise is hard work. It is much more costly to the body than movement. Over the course of this chapter you will learn to spot when your kids are lacking in exercise and how to improve their level of both activity and simple movement over the course of the day, every day.

To illustrate the key difference between movement and exercise, think of someone in your circle of acquaintances who is always moving, who cannot sit still and as a result never puts on weight. They expend energy all day long by fidgeting, standing up instead of sitting down, running up stairs when they could as easily have walked. These are the same people who struggle to keep their weight up at a normal level. They tend not to store energy, they use it instead. They may never have darkened the door of a gym; they do not necessarily go for a walk in the park every day: in truth, they don't need to in order to keep their weight under control. They have their energy expenditure at maximum capacity at all times. This is also represented by the child who cannot sit still. That child generally has no weight issues. The movers and shakers among us tend not to be bothered with overweight.

You will also know someone in your sphere who can do nothing but sit still. They seem never to move, only perhaps when pushed to it out of sheer necessity. When they do move, watching it can feel like watching a movie in slow motion. Every move seems measured and controlled: speed never seems to be involved. These are the same people who tend always to battle to keep their weight under control. They might have been heavy as a child and now they are heavy as an adult, as they tend to store energy in their fat cells instead of spending it. Children who are slow to spend energy tend towards overweight, unless their calorie intake is kept to a moderate amount and they are kept active. These are the kids who will tend to put on weight over the Christmas, Hallowe'en or Easter break, when they are allowed free rein over their stash of sweets and chocolate eggs. Their system is very efficient at storing fat, instead of expending that energy. I am the first to admit that we are all different: some of us are movers and some of us are not; and so it is for your kids, their cousins, their friends.

We are all born different. Of this I have no doubt. I see the evidence every day I work with clients. Some lose weight very easily and are energised to do so, while for others it feels like pulling teeth: slow, laborious and painful is how they might describe their weight-loss journey. So we move differently. As children, some of us were slow-moving, while others found it difficult to sit still for even a moment. As adults, we can spot the difference.

Yes, inherently you may be measured and slow-moving, but you can choose to be a 'mover and a shaker'. You can choose to run up the stairs instead of pressing the button on the lift again and again in the hope of saving yourself the journey. You can choose to walk around with vim and vigour; choose to go to the rest room at work that is two flights of stairs or three blocks away (if you think you will get away with it). You do not need to circle the door of the supermarket like a hawk, in the hope of getting a parking space right by the trolley bay. Park as far away as possible and walk. Look for opportunities for movement in your day. Embrace such opportunities. We should not avoid movement, we should relish it. In no time at all, you will be the one who always dashes out to get the newspaper in the afternoon, having cancelled the delivery; you pop out to school on foot, in all weathers; you plan outdoor weekend activities, weather notwithstanding. You have become that 'mover' who was always waiting to be released from captivity within your sedentary self.

You can also get your children to move more. They need to be taught this. Remember, we teach mainly by example. Why not walk to school on days that you can manage it, perhaps only once a week to begin with? Maybe walking home from school is a more achievable target.

This will not suit everyone, of course, but certainly on the weekends, when our time is our own, we should aim to get out of the house more, with our children in tow. We should certainly walk to the shop on a Sunday to get the 'Sunday treat', or to sports training if it is nearby. Equally, we should walk around the pitch with the other kids while watching one of them training; or perhaps that half hour you spend with one of them every Saturday in the car while waiting for another could be better spent walking briskly round the block. Of course, this means a little organisation, in terms of suitable coats, hats and shoes, but it is well worth while. If you are not motivated to do this yourself, you have little hope of getting your kids to do it for themselves. I always see this as a cart-before-the-horse scenario. By this I mean that we need to be out there, getting wet, getting sweaty – and perhaps muddy – first, before we in fact *want* to do it again. On a wet day it is a very hard 'sell' to expect any one of your kids to get out of the car, until you enjoy your first outing together. Of course, bribery may initially need to be part of the equation: if you promise to have a 'movie night' later the first time, the next time it will be a far easier 'sell'. Try it. No amount of words on paper can convince you of this until you put it into action yourself and *feel* the benefits. It might seem a slightly illogical argument; that getting your kids wet and muddy in the name of exercise is worth the cleaning-up operation afterwards. But when you and they both feel invigorated, instead of lethargic, at the end of such an outing, you will begin to look forward to embracing activity the next time.

Many of us parent our kids so well these days that the activities we bring them to and from are often the primary focus of our leisure time, and I often think we might be overdoing it. 'Over-parenting', as I like to call it, might be a recent phenomenon that is partly responsible for our kids getting fatter. You know the routine: you are dropping one child off to piano lessons while the other does their homework in the car; or you are sweating blood and tears in the tiny cubicle at swimming lessons, week after week, drying one child's hair while the other one is hell bent on making their way into the swimming pool fully clad! And all for a thirty-minute lesson, during which your child chats and half listens to the instructor for the most part of the class, and is perished with cold by the end of it. Is this exercise? Barely! This is learning a new skill. For many kids, this is not the hour of exercise we need to get them to achieve every single day. It is a far cry from it.

Exercise is very different from movement. You know you are exercising when your heart rate is up, when your lungs are expanding and breathing is harder. It is that simple to spot. Your kids are exercising when they are playing chase, not necessarily when they are pottering around the swimming pool. They get exercise from walking the dog – as long as the dog is not the boss and stops to leave its mark on everything that isn't tied down. They get exercise also, of course, when they play sports such as athletics, football, gymnastics, volleyball and the likes, especially when playing in a match. Our younger kids really only get exercise through play. In short, encourage your kids to play more. Send them out of the house. They all, at every age, need a full one hour of exercise per day. No exceptions. Do your kids achieve this daily hour of out-of-breath activity?

> Can you remember being told as a child, 'Go out and play'?

Why are we so afraid these days to let our kids out of the house? I am not sure. Yes, we are busier than ever. Perhaps we are not always at home to be there in case something happens to them. We are at home on some days of the week, though. On these days, at the very least, encourage your kids to go out. No: *send* them out. Can you remember being told as a child, 'Go out and play'? I certainly can recall that mantra. Of course television was not a feature of our day. We were allowed to watch *Sesame Street* on a Saturday morning – only if it was not a beautifully sunny day outside – and that was it. Old as I might sound, I'm not that old. It was not that long ago.

Nowadays our fool-proof babysitter is the television, any time of the day or night. *We* need to have the discipline to turn off the television and to send our children out to play. 'Go out and play before dinner' should be your mantra. We need the discipline to carry this out and insist on it. Yes, they will moan and groan sometimes. That is part of the job description of parenting, as you well know. In time, they will get used to playing outside more, and the good news is that it is contagious. When your kids go out on their bikes, their roller blades or with a football, the others in the neighbourhood will soon join them – they simply cannot resist. Trust me on this.

> Nowadays our fool-proof babysitter is the television, any time of the day or night. We need to have the discipline to turn off the television and to send our children out to play. 'Go out and play before dinner' should be your mantra.

In the playground you might notice that in recent years we have taken to playing *for* our children. Have you found yourself doing this? You will see the well-meaning mum or dad chasing after their child for fear of seeing them fall, or holding their hand on a climbing frame when, in fact, the child is more than capable of climbing it unaided. We mean well when we stand below them, just in case they slip off, but the result is often the whining, helpless 'look at me, look at me' child who should instead be off interacting with others of their own age, making friends and building up a head of steam, having fun playing. This used to be the case in the past. If you were lucky enough to be brought to a playground, you played. Your parents dropped you off. You played with children, not with adults. Let your children play. They instinctively know how to, it is good for them – and you can benefit from the break. Perhaps you could get into the habit of walking around the internal perimeter of the playground while doing your time there, in a bid to get yourself moving more.

I recently attended a parent–teacher meeting where one of my children's teacher visibly grimaced in horror at the notion that at home our kids are allowed to run around the house and jump on sofas, on a wet day. She thought I was quite mad, I'm sure. My point to her was that it is important to our family that our children can get rid of their pent-up energy, every single day of the week, whether after school or on a long wet Sunday indoors.

We are kinetic beings. This means that we were designed for movement. As you may know, some species of shark can never stay still; if they do, they die. While this may be a slightly exaggerated comparison, I genuinely feel that we are all happier when we are moving. Our kids love to move. They deserve it. Of course, as a result of this approach, my house is not pristine; but in my mind it is better parenting to prioritise their health, physical and mental, than to bring them to every organised activity known to humankind. Yes, many activities are very worthwhile. The skills learned during them are a very important part of growing up. Simple play is also a great stimulant for kids, though, and should not be overlooked. Children bond with each other through play (of course they fight, too): they get scenario games going, in which they put on all available coats and hats and go to Antarctica (the attic room) on an expedition; or they play Transformers, chasing each other around the kitchen counter-top; or they are rugby tackling each other; or pretending to be spies. The sky's the limit when and if your children are allowed free rein at home, within reason of course.

Needless to say, I have no china on display in my house; no valuable artefacts; no delicate pieces of furniture. As I see it, this is *their* house as much as it is mine – in fact more so, when I think of how formative a role it will have in their development. I can look forward to getting the china on display in my retirement!

I strongly recommend trying perhaps to lessen the activities load for a term or two if you feel your child might be overdoing it. Try this as an experiment to see the impact it has on your child, to let them get creative and energised about their free time. All kids deserve free time, and plenty of it. It not only gets them using energy, but it fuels their creativity and imagination too.

Energy spent means calories spent. The WHO tells us that adults need to take ten thousand steps a day for health. This is what I would categorise as movement. What does ten thousand steps a day look like? Taking my own working day as an example, I can do no more than a poor two and a half thousand steps if I see clients from nine to five. I rarely do this, but I have occasionally done so while wearing a pedometer, to see what the numbers looked like. Not good! If I am off on, say, a Monday, when I run around like a headless chicken, catching up on supermarket shopping, activities, housework, I can achieve a mere seven and a half thousand steps. Why so few? In reality, my car does most of the work. If, weather permitting, I play tennis on a Monday night I will get my ten thousand steps completed. The point I am making here is that it is a lot harder for us to get our required steps completed, per day, unless we are putting a concerted effort into it. A young nurse walking the wards and up and down stairs in a large hospital, though, will quite easily achieve his or her quota. I get people to move more in their workplaces by walking and talking instead of emailing the person in the office next door. Get off your seat more at work. Be the person who goes out to get the milk at break time or who never emails in-house, who instead drops into that person's office. You may laugh, but we do this. In a previous working life, I used to regularly email the person next door to me. Daft!

It is the same for our children. They need opportunities in their day to move more and expend energy. Their working day might include their crèche, playschool, or school day. While on some days they may get outdoor playtime, it is not necessarily going to happen every day and they are quite often not allowed to run in the yard, due to concerns for others' safety. They still, however, need to incorporate plenty of movement into that day. They need to expend the amount of calories that they took in that day, and more if you are hoping for their waistbands to loosen.

When your child is older, send them out to get the milk at the garage, on foot or by bike. Get your kids to walk the dog, make their own beds, bring their uniform upstairs when they have changed after school, bring their books downstairs for return to the library, brush the floor, vacuum the carpet, put clothes on the line, weed the garden with you. You get the idea. When our children are small they love these jobs. They feel very grown up doing them. These are valuable lessons for them to learn: that jobs are part of everyday family life; that movement is normal; that watching the television is a treat for when the jobs are done; that being outdoors, in all weathers, is good for health.

I recently updated our family's wet-weather gear for very little money in one of our great cheap supermarkets. For the price of one child's winter coat I got all six of us suited and booted in lightweight wet-weather gear. The fun is mighty when you get everyone out on a wet and windy day. From howling wind and rain, to muddy puddles, to feeding ducks and kicking leaves, kids of all ages (adults too) feel liberated and happy to be out in the elements and in touch with nature, instead of watching television in super-heated houses. After a walk in the elements the treat can be a packet of crisps and glass of cordial in the pub. Having earned the 'Sunday treat', as it is called in our house, makes you value it all the more as a child and then later as an adult.

My seventh rule has to be, in all its simplicity: **GET MOVING!** Stop avoiding movement; embrace it. Look for opportunities for movement in your child's day. If you instill good habits now – always walking, skipping, running for yourself – instead of expecting to be ferried from A to B and delivered to the front door of a host of activities, your child will be much more likely to be active for life. It amazes me that we have come, in so short a time, to the point that our kids can demand mobile phones from the age of eight, in the name of security or independence, yet we will not let them out of our sight to go and play, climb trees, explore, even when they are in possession of the all-important mobile. Our kids need play, they enjoy play, they have to be allowed to get out more and play.

Exercise, as I mentioned earlier, is quite different from movement. When we exercise we can feel our heart beating and we get out of breath. When this happens we expand our lungs and use our all-important heart muscle, and both organs benefit greatly from the exertion. This is the basis of aerobic fitness.

Our children require such fitness for health, regardless of their weight. If they need to get to a healthier weight, exercise also uses up excess energy, which, in combination with better eating habits, as outlined in this book, gets quick and easy results. As a child I can remember having to walk to the creamery every day to get milk. I might have been only five years old, but the pace set by the adult with me was such that I had to run about three steps for every one of her strides. Exercise for a child does not need to be more complicated than that (nor does it for an adult, incidentally).

I am of the opinion that introducing children to the gym as a means of getting them to exercise is akin to punishment. Most adults have a love–hate relationship with the gym: either we love it and frequent it regularly for weeks; or we cannot stand the sight of the gym bag and secretly hope to forget to put it in the car boot so as to have the excuse we were looking for not to go to the gym in the first place. Our children can do without going to the gym: they do not deserve to be punished with exercise machinery that could eat them up.

Instead, take them to the park and throw a ball with them: you know you do not want to be in the gym with them either, or indeed in the car outside waiting for them. If you are a member of a tennis club, for example, bring them along and let them attempt to play with you, or to be the ball boy or girl at your game. Send a small child outside with bubbles and allow them to run daftly around after them. When I was taking three steps for every one adult stride at the age of five, I was out of breath: therefore I was getting aerobic exercise.

Have you ever chased one of your kids around the kitchen table for fun? If you have, I guarantee you were momentarily out of breath. Kids are fast, and they corner a lot better than we do! Even allowing your children to run around the kitchen, playing chase, is allowing them to get some of their daily dose of aerobic activity. **Our kids need one hour of aerobic exercise every day.** Do yours achieve this?

The recommended one hour of exercise can be broken into three or four parts for your child, to make it more practical, if necessary. For instance, in a day, your child might have had two ten-minute play sessions (hopefully of an active nature) at school; they might have played chase inside (go on, let them) for ten minutes after homework; and you might briskly walk to the shop later on to get bread for tomorrow's lunch and drop them off to play outside, with their friends, on the way home. In all, they should, with your guidance, have achieved well over the requisite hour's activity by the end of business that day.

Compare this to the not so unusual scenario of your child coming home to be allowed to watch television straight away for an hour or more, then finding that they have to address themselves to their homework before it gets too late and they are too cranky. At the end of this time you will notice that it is probably close to dinner time and any other children playing outside have gone inside for their evening meal. After dinner it might be dark, or nearly dark, so you would prefer your child to remain indoors, at which time they play either on the computer or on the hand-held equivalent for an hour. This hour of inactivity is followed by another hour of television before bed. This may seem a slightly exaggerated case: to be honest it is not. It is very easy, if your eye is not constantly on the ball, to allow this scenario to develop. Total inactivity is the result. As a result of this approach our kids become lazy, through no fault of their own. It is our responsibility to get them moving and exercising. We do not want unfit children, surely. In the example detailed above, your child would be much less likely to stay inside, stock still and entranced by whatever gadget they are allowed to play with, if the rules in your house stated that they are allowed only half an hour gadget time, after playing outside (or indoors, actively, on a wet day) for an hour. Television time should also be restricted to their favourite programme only, not passively watching whatever is on at whatever time they get the notion to switch it on.

Our children need to be taught that being active is normal. In the days when the nobility were people of leisure and excessive exertion was frowned upon, people believed that we are born with a certain amount of energy to expend in our lifetime. Therefore, if people were wealthy enough not to have to labour in the fields, the most exercise they tended to take was a turn about the room during an evening by the fire, chatting or reading (think *Pride and Prejudice*). They did their best to conserve energy in the hope of living longer, and pitied the poor workers who had to toil and expend their energy reserves daily and thus died younger. They were wrong. We are, in fact, made of exactly the opposite stuff. We were made to move.

We are kinetic beings. **We thrive when we move.** The more we exercise and move, the fitter we are. Generally speaking, the fitter you are, the longer you tend to live (if all goes according to plan). We certainly need to get this message across to our kids. This current generation of adults has become rapidly more sedentary than probably the eighteenth-century gentry ever were, when you take into account how long we spend each day in the car, behind a desk and in front of the television. Our children cannot be expected to be active, going into adulthood, if we ourselves are not active. We need to first remind ourselves that being active is meant to be the norm and our kids will, as always, learn by example.

Rule 9:
Just portion control it

If you have read this far you will have a good idea of the principles on which I base my arguments. But you are still convinced that while these rules might work for other kids, they will fail for yours. Your kids are the exception. No one has ever met a child as picky as yours. The theory might be fine, but in all practicality you believe you have no hope of getting your child to even try any new approaches to food. **Be patient.** Be patient most of all with yourself.

When you yourself are convinced, you will have the conviction of your beliefs to push forward with your new food agenda. I have met plenty of picky kids: kids who will not eat anything green; kids who run a mile when they see any kind of herb in their dinner; kids who will not sit down to eat; kids who have odd rules about food. I've seen the lot. Your kids as well as mine can be very picky indeed.

Have you ever noticed how after any sickness your child's appetite for strong-tasting foods will have diminished and they will favour bland food such as toast, ice cream, crackers, milk and biscuits? It always takes a week or two, even more, for me to get any of mine back on track to liking strongly flavoured foods again, such as curry or fish cakes or oily fish. Their instinct is to keep things bland, so that they can maximise calories (in the form of ice cream and cake) and thus recover faster. If you allow this newly found liking for all things bland to stick, you will end up with a child with a very limited repertoire of foods that are acceptable to them. We need to push their boundaries for them, as they do not generally look for change themselves: kids tend to dislike change of any sort. So, if your child has ever been sick, you may have unwittingly allowed them to stick to a very narrow range of foods because they obviously prefer them.

Given the chance, however, your child will keep on narrowing down this repertoire, if so inclined, until they like only potato waffles and sausages! You may laugh, but this is not as daft as it may at first seem. I have met plenty of children whose food repertoire is not much broader than this: it may be just pasta and cheese for dinner, every day. While a particular food might not be harmful in itself, it is important to realise that a child will never allow themselves to starve, when in an environment of plenty. They will always get enough calories to give themselves enough energy to complete their day. They can, however, miss out on fibre and a plethora of nutrients if stuck in a food rut, while simultaneously taking in inordinate amounts of salt and fat (as in the sausages and waffles example). We can do a lot better than this for our kids' nutritional status.

Kids need to be able to eat whatever they want, within reason. **There is no such thing as a bad food.** A single processed waffle will not harm your child. There is no one food that is better than all the rest. Getting your child to eat the 'super-food' blueberries will not, of itself, give them a healthy diet. There is more to it than that. There is balance. Blueberries are one of many sources of valuable antioxidant nutrients, not the only one and not the best. At their price I would need some alternatives! Think colour. What would stain your child's clothes as fast as a squashed blueberry? Beetroot would, for instance. All coloured berries are good, all coloured vegetables and fruit contain plentiful supplies of the antioxidants our kids need to thrive. I will admit that it would be very ambitious to expect your little ones to eat pickled beetroot from a jar, but many are happy to eat the plain vacuum-packed ones (I have very rarely boiled my own beetroot) as part of a salad lunch.

Bite-sized foods inherently appeal to kids, because they can pick food up, sniff, poke and generally interact with new foods before considering eating them. I often do a summertime salad, set out on the table, that includes such foods as beetroot in one bowl, tiny tomatoes in another, chopped boiled egg in another, lettuce leaves, chopped spring onion, tuna mayonnaise, cucumber sticks, carrot sticks, etc. The kids sit at the table, each with a wrap on their plate. They can make up their sandwich according to their particular taste. I might, on occasion, nudge them to try new things, but I find they are quite happy to do it themselves when presented with choice – over time, of course, not all in one day. One tends to be the most adventurous, then another competes with the first, and I need to do little more than sit there and enjoy my own wrap.

If you aim for perfection and expect everything to be tried and eaten in one sitting, I'm sorry to tell you that you will be disappointed. When we aim for perfection we are doomed to failure! The middle ground is what I am always aiming for when it comes to my children's relationship with food. Yes, they will eat lots of different foods: not all foods, and some more than others. But they also eat plenty of 'treat' foods and even 'rubbish' foods, for example at Hallowe'en, or at a birthday party. **For our kids to have a normal relationship with food, I think it is important that we do not ban certain types of food.** They want to fit in with their friends and with the norm. Eating is a social activity, and it should be normal to eat whatever you want. 'Within reason' is what I hear myself add to this sentence as soon as I utter it.

The problem today is that the bar has been lowered considerably when it comes to food quality and our standards are bottoming out, especially when one looks at what foods are being marketed to our kids. Chocolate-covered space balls for breakfast do not represent good food to me. Double-decker pizzas with cheese-style filling in the crusts do not represent the makings of a balanced meal. Cracker and dip snacks for lunchboxes will not give our children much beyond fat and salt. Our kids need good food. However, even I can see a need to allow them a box of chocolate-covered space balls on their birthday weekend, for instance. I would not ban them: delay, delay, delay would be my motto. So the promise of chocolate-covered space balls can carry me through a good three weeks of complaining that they never get to eat anything like that, before I ever have to buy them. The good news then is that when they are gone they are gone!

> For our kids to have a normal relationship with food, I think it is important that we do not ban certain types of food. They want to fit in with their friends and with the norm. Eating is a social activity, and it should be normal to eat whatever you want. 'Within reason' is what I hear myself add to this sentence as soon as I utter it.

When it comes to hydrogenated and trans fats, though, I do draw the line, as far as I can. In my house you will not find foods containing hydrogenated fats. This takes a little effort, but it is well worth it. What are these fats? They are fats that have been damaged by food processing and by very high temperatures. Some resultant fats are termed trans fats (partially hydrogenated), as they have been transformed chemically from what they once were and have a 'bent' structure, chemically, as a result of the process they went through.

While these hydrogenated and partially hydrogenated or trans fats can be termed vegetable fats on a food label, and therefore sound like healthy fats, in fact they no longer resemble a vegetable fat in chemical terms. To produce these fats, hydrogen gas is pumped through vats of vegetable oil at extremely high temperature under extremely high pressure, in the presence of a heavy metal, usually a nickel catalyst, to produce hydrogenated fat (which we call margarine) or partially hydrogenated fats that contain trans fats. The structure of the vegetable fat is changed by the addition of hydrogen to the oil so that by the end of the process it does not resemble a vegetable fat, neither is it a natural animal fat: it is a manufactured version that lies somewhere between the two.

The reason why I allow butter and chocolate to be eaten aplenty in my house is that the science of saturated fats is very simple. If you eat some animal fat it is good for you: it follows natural pathways in the body that aid its digestion; and it can perform some bodily tasks. If you eat too much of it, it is stored in your body and can dangerously increase your blood cholesterol levels. Our children can, of course, have some butter, cheese, chocolate, mincemeat burgers; but if they eat too many of these they will store fat and thus will get fat. It is very straightforward science.

However, because hydrogenated fats are an artificial product, there are no natural pathways in the body to deal with them and they will be stored more readily.

We are seeing more and more evidence of this. The fat pad I referred to in Rule 1 is partly formed as a result of the intake of such poor-quality fats. The fat cells closest to the stomach get the goods first, in terms of excess energy, and they store that unnecessary fat fastest, resulting in the child with a waistband inappropriate for their age and height. It is that easy. **Hydrogenated and partially hydrogenated fats are bad for our children's health.** Such processed fat does them no good. It is actively bad for them.

Denmark has banned trans fats from sale. I love that. We need to open our eyes to see how harmful our current approach to our kid's nutrition can be. If you have observed the ferocity with which advertising campaigns are directed at our children you will have to admit that we are not stringent enough, by any means, about what we allow our kids to be sold on. In my house, the kids are only allowed to watch television if the sound is muted during the ad breaks. We are killing our kids with kindness by allowing them to demand whatever they fancy. Many snack foods directed for sale at our kids contain large amounts of hydrogenated fats. Such ingredients are used to benefit the profit margins of manufacturers. They are not included in food to benefit the health of our children. Hydro-genated fats came into common use by manufacturers in the 1940s because they are a cheaper alternative to butter, not because the industry was looking for a healthy alternative. Margarine is bad for us. It has been proven to have a negative impact on our immune system. It not only makes our kids fat; it also makes them sick. Butter, by comparison, is good for them, in moderation. Butter contains two ingredients, at most: cream and salt. That is how I like the ingredients lists on my food labels – nice and short.

Where do we find hydrogenated fat (margarine)? In almost all commercially produced biscuits, cakes, scones, biscuit bars, tarts, pastries, crumbles, desserts and savoury pies, unless stated otherwise. Margarine or vegetable fat is mainly used by manufacturers for reasons of economy and profit. The reason you are charged considerably more for an 'all-butter' pastry tart is that butter is a more expensive ingredient and you have to pay the difference. When baking at home I use butter. The result is as high in fat as the margarine-containing equivalent, but the quality is superior and so is the taste. Of course, manufacturers are always evolving their product range and they do respond to market demands. As a result, you might recently have noticed labelling that highlights 'no hydrogenates'. This is a great new trend. We need to raise our awareness of such issues and in time the manu-facturers will meet our demands. If it becomes clear that we are willing to pay a little more for the 'all-butter' equivalent, it will be made more commonly available and as a result will come down in price, as a result of the economy of scale.

We all love a bargain, so we feel we should not have to pay any more than necessary for a product. I think we need to raise the bar a little. If we buy processed foods we need to buy good-quality versions and pay a little extra for them. I have had to ban my mother from bringing cheap and cheerful multi-packs of bars and biscuits for the kids. She loves a bargain. While she meant well, I just did not feed these bars to the children. Eventually she got the message. I needed to spell out the problem with something costing too little in 'you get what you pay for' terms. And this is the same woman who only buys organic vegetables! Nowadays she often brings organic fruit and perhaps garlic, just because she knows we use it a lot and of course it would have been on offer in the supermarket, but she also brings good-quality milk chocolate, and that's fine. Simple chocolate is a good food. Kids love chocolate. It is no hardship for them to eat chocolate instead of a biscuit bar. Again, list the ingredients in chocolate – it is pretty easy: cocoa mass, sugar, cocoa butter, cocoa powder, emulsifier, natural flavouring. About six ingredients is a good indication of quality in this case. When it reads like a chemistry set, you know you are in cheap and not so cheerful territory.

What about the dreaded children's birthday party? These can range from the 'uber-cautious' rice cake and fruit fest to the more common chicken nugget and curly fries extravaganza – with every sticky coloured sweet known to humankind, for the sheer 'free-for-all' of it. How do we hope to cope with our child who might be prone to over-eating on such an occasion? How, further, do we get them to achieve balance on that day?

Well, my advice would be to simply allow them to have what they like at the party, and not to worry too much. If you tell your child to restrict their intake at the party, you are either barking up the wrong tree, or you are setting your child up to feel confused and anxious on the day, neither of which achieves a good result. Be careful to use the language of fun around such food-centred occasions. Tell them to have fun, to enjoy playing with their friends and to enjoy having their tea with friends. If you feel certain that your child will eat far too many sweets, gently remind them not to get themselves full to the point of feeling sick. There is bound to have been an occasion in the past when one of the kids got sick after a family gathering or similar occasion, and this can serve as a very simple and direct reminder of what not to do.

In our house we have numerous reminders on which we can call. 'Remember when you threw up into three bedrooms after the baby's christening?' is one such reminder I used for years on my eldest, when she was learning how to navigate her way through the kiddies' party scene! She remembered how horrible that felt and as a result learned how to contain herself at such a do. When your child comes home after the party you might ask them, 'Did you have your tea?', 'Did you enjoy it?', 'Did you have some lovely cake?', 'Was it a princess cake?', 'Would you like a cake like that for your next birthday?' In other words, be open and direct about what they consumed; keep it fun and light, then realise that yes, they have eaten lots of 'junk' today. So be it. They do not now need to have dinner with the rest of the family on this occasion, as they will have already eaten. Instead, later on, when it might be time for a bed-time snack, they will benefit from fruit and plenty of it, as it is one component of their day they will certainly have missed out on. Perhaps you could give them some stewed apple and custard, or some milk and a banana.

Daily balance is our goal. If, for reasons beyond your control, it cannot be achieved on a particular day, think about the overall balance of the week as a whole. Perhaps your child is old enough to have a sleep-over at a friend's house and is allowed all sorts of freedoms there you would not allow at home, such as midnight feasts and the like. The following day I would instantly start thinking about kids' curry with extra vegetables and baby cucumbers in their lunchbox. Neurotic as this may sound, it works!

If you do not achieve this kind of balance you will find that your kids start complaining of constipation (as a sick tummy, often) which is really something no child should ever suffer. They have a good strong digestion at this age that should be kept freely moving with an adequate fibre intake (fruit, vegetables and whole foods). The growing incidence of bowel cancer – which results from lack of fibre in the diet – is a concern for all of us. We need to protect our kids against running the risk of bowel cancer later on in life.

When my oldest child goes to the cinema with friends on a Sunday afternoon, I ensure, every time, that we have a vegetable-based meal in the middle of the day. In place of dessert or the 'Sunday treat' she gets some pocket money, with which she can go off and buy some sweets after the movie. More often, she uses the money to buy a little trinket and only spends a little on sweets. What's great about this is that she can have her cake and eat it too, in terms of treat and trinket. The choice is hers, and kids love having some autonomy as they get older. The cinema should really be treat enough in its own right.

If you like to bake it is a great idea to get your children involved in this activity. It is much more fun than play dough, in my opinion, and the clean-up is

KILKENNY COUNTY LIBRARY

much easier too. **Involve your child in food preparation.** Let them make some choices when it comes to food. You very likely have some child-friendly cookbooks at home that they can trawl through and become inspired to make chocolate crisp bars or the like. This is good. It gets them to make and do and understand that food is a good thing, a fun thing – and best of all, you get to lick the bowl and eat the spoils. Straightforward wholemeal scones, if you make them with a small scone cutter so that they come out of the oven high and fluffy, are a real winner. If you freeze some after they cool, you have ready-made lunchbox fillers for the following week. Is there a child out there who would not like a flapjack at snack time? Yes, it is extremely high in fat and sugar, but when looked at properly it is a good wholesome treat: it also contains oats, and when it is made with butter, not margarine, it contains only good-quality fats. And it is of far superior quality to a shop-bought biscuit bar.

Kids feel empowered by being able to prepare part of their own meals. The result of regular involvement in food preparation – say you allow Saturday afternoon to be 'baking day' – is that in no time at all your child will want to peel the carrots on a Tuesday and wash the potatoes on a Thursday. I can attest to this. We need to give our kids some ownership of their diet. They may want volcano potatoes three days running (this is what we call mashed potatoes with baked beans flowing down the mountain), but you could add money (sliced carrot 'coins') one day, trees (you guessed it – broccoli) the next, lava rocks (peas) the next, to accompany their favourite. Ask them, 'Would you like carrot money or broccoli trees with your volcano today?'

This approach works when they are small, of course: you are the boss but they get an element of choice. Add to that the freedom of choosing Saturday's dessert and actually making it themselves and you have kids who are happy to eat their dinner that day. I will guarantee it. Just recently my eight-year-old boy made beef stew for the whole family using a recipe in a children's cookbook. The reason I mention this is that he, in fact, is the one who has moved furthest away from involvement in the kitchen of late. He does not bake a whole lot any more (the two smaller kids have taken up the mantle) and while he will set the table for mealtime, under duress, he tends to be too busy doing other things to spend his time on boring old baking. All that prompted him, in this instance, to make Saturday's dinner was a cake sale in his school the previous week. He and his little brother made muffins with orange icing (as he had for years previously) for the sale – under my supervision – and suddenly he was inspired to make dinner the following weekend. He took two books away with him and came back declaring beef stew was going to be his offering on Saturday. I just pottered on the day while to my amazement he peeled and chopped onion and garlic and carrot and leek and potato (I bought the beef chopped). He not only made a meal everyone loved, but it took two hours to cook in the oven so it did not seem labour-intensive to the boy who went off to play for the rest of the afternoon. I did not see that coming. I was very pleasantly surprised. He told me that he wanted to be able to cook dinner when he grows up and moves out of home! A great result for everyone.

If you allow your children to have some control over what they eat, so that they feel free to choose, not dictated to, then they really can get to eat whatever they want (within reason). My rule on this approach, rule number nine, is: **JUST PORTION CONTROL IT.** Your children's health does not depend on their getting so-called 'super foods' every day, nor is it detrimental to their health to allow them to eat 'rubbish' every now and again. Balance is what we are after. **Keep foods good quality, wholesome and tasty for the most part and the odd digression will not add up to a whole lot of damage.** I think the French approach to food, the motto that goes something like 'a little of what you fancy does you good', is a great simplification of this approach. It does not matter if, on a rare occasion, your child eats chocolate-covered space balls for breakfast. It matters a lot, however, if we allow these sugar-laden, nutrient-devoid concoctions to be a regular feature of our child's diet, in place of nutritious options such as porridge, muesli or wholemeal bread.

So let's say that your child is now of an age that they simply will not eat what you would like them to. Where do you begin to make changes? Initially I would suggest that you get them looking through child-friendly cookbooks, either on their own or with your guidance. You should get plenty of ideas, all of which will be of good nutrient quality, from these books. Yes, your child will immediately flick to the dessert pages: no surprise there. They can choose a dessert to make, of course, that will be eaten after the main course. As for the main course, there should be no limits: only that you may need to go out later and buy the ingredients. I suggest, in this initial phase of making changes, that you might bring the child with you to the shop. You will have your list of ingredients: you might also ask them to buy some fruit they like and their favourite vegetable and this can be followed by a trip to the dessert ingredients aisle. Once the dinner has been made and dessert eaten you will find you have one new addition to the menu for the week. This sounds simplistic, but often the best ideas are simple. Build one new dinner into the repertoire of dishes you cook per week and in seven weeks' time you will have a new dinner a day. Yes, there will be hiccups along the way, but it is very worthwhile to make the effort.

As for your child's penchant for cheap and nasty processed foods (long tubular containers of potato crisps come instantly to mind), I would suggest you wean them off the really poor versions of these and on to less processed versions. Remember to portion control their intake of such treat foods. Turn the long tubular disaster-zone into an old-fashioned packet of crisps like the ones we all ate as children. With approximately 150kcal per smaller packet this does none of the damage that a 900kcal tube can do by comparison, when there is a free-for-all approach to snacks in the house. Give them what they want, a little of what they want, when they have done their best with today's breakfast, lunch and dinner. They will have earned it and so will you.

Rule 10:

Have a strategy

The day never holds as many surprises as we think it might. I am often told by a client that they had to take an unexpected flight or a train journey during a particular week, which threw their eating plans out enough that they had to eat on the hoof. After buying a rubbery old ham sandwich or missing a meal, they will have ended up snacking from the mini-bar of a hotel out of necessity, brought on by unexpected hunger and cravings late in the day. We are often under the impression that we are too busy to buy and prepare food on every occasion and we can feel especially helpless when it comes to exceptions to our normal routine.

I would argue that the twenty-four hours ahead generally do not hold as many unexpected events as we may think. In most cases, if we have to go to a meeting in another city, or take an extended journey with the kids, we plan a few days ahead. When we are preparing for any such journey, we should prepare in terms of meals as much as we would in terms of clothes and the personal items we could not live without. I can guarantee you that you would never embark on such a journey without your wallet or purse and mobile phone. Why, therefore, would you leave your food options to chance? The chances of finding good food on trains or at airports are slim. It always amazes me that in Paris, for instance, one can get the freshest, tastiest, most scrumptious almond croissant imaginable at a pâtisserie en route to the airport, but as soon as you cross the threshold of the airport the croissants are of a calibre found in any supermarket around the world: in other words, they are very poor indeed.

When we are serious about the quality of food that we allow to pass our lips and those of our kids, we need to take responsibility for the entire day's eating, whatever the circumstances. I have a 'nine out of ten' rule when it comes to food. If you do your best and achieve what we have set out to do in this book, nine times out of ten, then the odd exception to the rule is just that: it is an aberration. This in itself is not a problem: it will not throw your balanced eating off by much.

It is when we have a 'making it up as we go along' approach to food that we run into trouble. You will be consistently disappointed at the calibre of foods available for kids out and about in the real world. After all your efforts at home, preparing good-quality, tasty foods that your kids now eat in moderate portions, you do not want to throw away all reason just because you are on a two-week holiday, for instance. Where in a restaurant or deli (outside Mediterranean Europe) would you find child-friendly fruit and salad dishes? They are certainly not as prominent as the sausage rolls or white, margarine-laden ham sandwiches you will readily find at every turn. Even when you do come across a salad that might, at a stretch, compete with the quick-fix option, it will never compare in attractiveness with the ever-appealing monstrous cookies, the muffin the size of your head (and twice that of your child's) or out-sized biscuit bar. Unless planned for, we really need to stay out of such shops, delis and restaurants. We are only human, after all. We can all fall prey to the warm, vanilla-scented, sugared air of such establishments. We see the monster muffin; we smell the frothy (and phenomenally expensive) coffee; we get to pick up the cereal bar before deciding whether to go for the 'healthier' choice than the slice of cake we actually desire (although the bar is in fact often higher in fat content than the cake).

While we may be able to rely (at least occasionally) on a little discipline so as not to indulge in the biggest muffin, the grandest coffee, along with a side of cream and the cereal bar, our kids cannot. They are, after all, children. They choose with their belly; they go for the largest, most chocolate-laden concoction, as we would ourselves, were we to allow ourselves to give in to such urges. You will, as a result of staying out of such establishments, save your family a fortune in calories (and cash).

We can, when necessary, easily and economically equip ourselves with all that we need for an entire day's eating by bringing our own lovingly prepared food for the journey. All of that Tupperware gathering dust at home in your cupboards needs to come out of storage. In fact, if we often travel with kids we need to get into the habit of never leaving home without it. As I have already said, kids thrive on routine. If you normally eat lunch at one o'clock, you should aim to have your picnic lunch at one o'clock. Keep to within one hour of your normal schedule if at all possible. In this example, lunch should never be later than two o'clock or earlier than twelve noon. If you stay on schedule, you will avoid hungry, whining kids and any resulting impulse eating at one end of the spectrum; and kids eating out of boredom, and thus overeating, at the other.

Have you ever noticed how much children love a picnic? Call anything you like a picnic and they get excited at the prospect of eating their food outdoors and on their lap. Whether you are pulling into a lay-by at the side of a motorway, eating at a wooden bench, or pulling out all the stops with a picnic basket and gingham tablecloth on a beach, call lunch a picnic. By attaching the notion of a picnic to any meal on the hoof you will get buy-in from kids of all ages and stages of life (and even parents and grandparents). Fun is what a picnic represents. Also involved is the notion of being allowed to eat casually and of having favourite foods to hand.

One of my kids' favourite picnic lunches when away for a week in an apartment, for example, is bread rolls bought in the local shop (the kids are not allowed out of the car!), ham and crisps. Once we've finished our mountain walk or we have declared it to be lunchtime, they make a ham and crisp roll. We do not take butter or mayonnaise in our back-pack, nor do we need to spend the money on (and acquire the calories of) a shop-bought, margarine- and mayonnaise-laden sandwich.

In the shop-bought version the margarine (which at home would be lovely, quality butter) goes on with a trowel, and another shovelful of mayonnaise is added. The amount of saturated fat and calories is building up before we even begin to consider fillers. Perhaps ham and coleslaw is your child's filling of choice. Huge amounts of mayonnaise-laden coleslaw will likely accompany the ham and we feel somewhat on track because it appears to contain vegetables, so we think it cannot be that bad. In fact, over ninety per cent of the calories in any regular coleslaw come from fat. Shocking, I know, but think about it. White cabbage and shredded carrot do not give you very many calories in comparison to full-fat mayonnaise. This is what you have put an effort into avoiding giving your child all week, only to let things slide, in the form of an innocent-looking sandwich, perhaps on a Sunday outing.

Don't get me wrong here. Kids need fat. Kids need to consume plenty of fat every day of the week. They need fat to perform essential tasks in the body, from making anti-inflammatory substances to building muscles and nerves to absorbing fat-soluble vitamins, along with many other essential functions. Kids' health will not thrive without fat. However, this fat needs to come, for the most part, from good-quality, fresh sources. In other words, fats that you can see. Simple as this principle may seem, it can be difficult enough to apply. Kids love processed, sugar-laden, high-fat foods, as we have discussed earlier. What they are not quite so keen on is plain boring old olive oil on a salad, with a little balsamic vinegar to balance it. Now that would be a hard sell for most kids I know. However, a teaspoon or two of mayonnaise on chopped boiled egg or tuna and sweetcorn seems to go down very well indeed with most.

'Why not the deli counter sandwich, then?' you may ask. Lack of necessary portion control is the answer. Two teaspoons of mayonnaise per person constitutes an appropriate amount of fat per sandwich. Either mayonnaise, perhaps, or coleslaw can be used, ideally not both. While fat is good for our children it contains 9kcals per gram and has to be used in consistent moderation in order to get our kids' weight back on track to being healthy. You do not know exactly how much fat there is in any pre-made or made-to-order sandwich unless you are right on top of the situation and, neurotic as it may sound, order 'No butter [because it is never butter, it is cheap margarine]; no mayo; no chips; no crisps; extra salad'! Then you pick up a sachet of mayonnaise, usually available on the counter (a humble two teaspoons per sachet) and use this to moisten an otherwise dry concoction. Portion control it!

In my family the smaller kids get a small bread roll and the older kids get a medium-sized one. It is always easy to lay your hands on a bottle of water for each person and fruit, too, is easy enough to find, if a shop is attached to the deli. Once I know that they have had a piece of fruit and an appropriately apportioned sandwich, they are also allowed to eat the 'holiday treat' of some sweets after lunch. After all, they will have been active all morning and will most likely spend the afternoon splashing about in the swimming pool, so they can do with the extra energy. On the odd occasion, then, when you have genuinely been taken by surprise and you find yourself unprepared, a stop-off at such a shop can still equip you with the basic ingredients for a good, balanced and fun meal. Now that you understand how lunch should look on the plate, to achieve a balanced meal, you will find you are no longer challenged on such occasions.

The proportions of the balanced plate must always (or nine times out of ten) be adhered to. I would, as far as possible, avoid altogether ready-made sandwich rolls from the deli counter when hoping to get the kids back on track to an appropriate number of calories per day. Ready-made in most cases means they do aim to kill you with kindness in a single sitting. What might be a sandwich at home turns into a bread-fest of enormous proportions at any deli counter.

You would be forgiven for thinking that I make these things up, but I can recall a recent visit to a deli while on mid-term break with the kids, when we stayed in an apartment in Kerry. While I was sourcing some good-quality ham to fill our rolls for what would constitute lunch on the top of Torc mountain (where the view is second only to a glimpse of heaven itself), I was struck dumb by the efforts of the deli staff at making sandwich rolls for other customers. I watched as one staff member put so much (poor-quality, rubbery) ham on a large bread roll that I couldn't help but tot up an approximate total of the calories the offending roll would eventually contain. Between handfuls of meat, piled high, poor-quality margarine aplenty, coleslaw and cheese, this monstrosity would have given its recipient a whopping 1,500kcals or so. There is not an active builder who can afford this many calories in one sitting and, besides, if a builder did consume that much he would, in all likelihood, prefer a quiet post-lunch nap to a productive afternoon's work.

In all seriousness, we seem to have lost the run of ourselves in recent years when it comes to portion control. If you went to a deli counter in France, for example, to buy a roll, what you might be presented with are such choices as bread (no butter, no mayonnaise, no coleslaw) with ham, bread with one slice of ham and one slice of cheese, bread with cheese only or bread with hard-boiled egg, tomato and lettuce. That's that. Spot the difference? It is not the fault of the deli counter staff member that they hand over a cholesterol-making bombshell to their customer, it is ours for accepting it. I personally could not give that to one of my kids. I (and they) would much rather the French-style roll, followed by a piece of fruit and then a packet of sweets or bar of chocolate. They get to eat lots of courses that are nutritious and portion-appropriate per person and I get to give them holiday treats, in the form of crisps and chocolate, so that they appreciate the reward for having completed a one-hour mountain walk and are re-energised for the descent. In this meal they get a fraction of the amount of fat, particularly saturated fat (the artery-hardening type) that would be contained in the pre-made sandwich.

You might notice that my kids are given crisps and chocolate. This would not happen, for instance, in a French child's normal day. For mine it means that I am ensuring they get plenty of fat for their day out. They only get these treats on occasions such as holidays. At home on a regular day, they would get fat in the form of a little butter or mayonnaise in their lunchtime sandwich.

Our kids need adequate fat intake on a regular daily basis; they have no requirement for artificially fat-free foods. Kids actually need to get approximately one-third of their daily calories from fat. This is a more generous amount than most of us would realise. We have fallen prey to the marketing by the fat-free brigade and to the notion that fat-free is the only acceptable way to eat. This is an utter fallacy. There is no science behind it. The sad fact of the matter is that when fat is taken out of what should be a reasonably high-fat product, say a cookie, sugar is usually used – in abundance – as a substitute. This sets our kids up for that blood sugar high, blood sugar low rollercoaster we discussed earlier, which has them constantly craving as a result. This is an unnecessary hardship. When allowed to eat one high-fat cookie your child will have a much better chance of feeling satisfied.

To put a number on it, your child would benefit from anywhere between approximately fifteen and thirty teaspoons of fat per day (depending on their size and activity level). Now if you could *see* every single teaspoon of fat in your child's intake during the day you would come to realise how generous this amount is. Clearly if your child needs to lose a large amount of body fat they do need to cut back considerably to the lower number on this scale, but under no circumstances should they cut out fat altogether. The problem is that we have no hope of identifying all the fat they consume during the day. They eat dairy products, eggs, breads, occasional chocolate or cakes, cookies, and prepared meals at home and outside the home. So you do not know the exact amount of fat they take in. When these foods are unprocessed, though, it is for the most part easy enough to get a handle on the amount consumed. We do not need to count fat-calories, ever: we need, instead, to allow some fat to be consumed at all meals, using moderation as our guide. We need to introduce our kids to such foods as oily fish (salmon, sardines, mackerel, trout) and raw nuts (four or five Brazil nuts at a time can be very satisfying) along with their more usual sources of fat, such as cheese, yoghurt, eggs, butter and olive oil (used in cooking). Variety is all-important here. They need, ideally, a 2:1 ratio of unsaturated fats to saturated fats for optimum health. How does this look?

Essentially they need saturated fats from such foods as dairy products (for calcium and good-quality protein along with the fat), eggs (containing the perfect protein) and butter (to make their bread taste good) with – occasionally – sausages, home-made burgers and chocolate or good-quality (ideally, home-made) cakes. What kids do not benefit from are fat-free versions of these. Kids do not want (nor should we) an egg white omelette. The yolk of the egg contains some very valuable nutrients as well as a little (beneficial) fat and cholesterol.

The other two-thirds of their fat intake should come mainly from nut and seed oils (sunflower, grape, canola, walnut, etc.); oily fish (salmon with ketchup, sardines on toast); olive oil (according to the WHO, we should frequently choose olive oil); and raw nuts and seeds. In short, sources where the oil is of good quality and has not been toasted, roasted or salted. If your child consumes oily fish once or twice per week, frequently eats nuts and/or seeds as an afternoon snack or in a good-quality bread (the rationale behind my bread recipe in Rule 7) and you use olive oil in preference to other oils in cooking and dressing meals at home, your child will get adequate unsaturated fats every day. This, in combination with daily consumption of dairy products and up to eight eggs per week, with only occasional high-fat meats (sausages, burgers) and treats, will ensure adequate fat nutrition. This means that your child will not crave those high-fat 'junk' foods they may have been constantly hounding you for when you previously tried to cut out fat, when in fact what they were looking for was a regular source of the all-important nutrient: fat.

So now that you have realised that perhaps your attempts at lowering your child's intake of fat were ever so slightly misguided you now need to shop according to your new requirements. You need to have a strategy. Your strategy must be straight-forward. Your child should get approximately 55–60% of their calories from carbohydrate every day, approximately 30% from fat and 12–15% from protein, with adequate fibre being provided through choosing mostly whole foods for the carbohydrates.

How do we achieve this consistently, every day? By going to the shop and buying the right food, in the correct proportions. While this answer may seem trite, shopping is what it all boils down to, in my experience. Those who develop a foolproof strategy when it comes to having the right foods available at the right time are always prepared and get the most consistent weight-loss results in my practice. **Preparation is an essential part of making a successful behaviour change.** To be prepared I use a list (but then I would!). My recommended shopping list, as you read earlier, includes fresh foods, tinned, frozen and long-life (dried). To further this strategic approach to shopping and food preparation I also have a life-saving ten-minute rule when it comes to food preparation – nine times out of ten, that is.

> Shopping is what it all boils down to, in my experience. Those who develop a foolproof strategy when it comes to having the right foods available at the right time are always prepared and get the most consistent weight-loss results.

I need to know that dinner, or lunch, takes no more than ten minutes of my time to get on the table most days of the week. Yes, I can do a labour-intensive smoked salmon quiche on a Sunday or for a special occasion, starting by making the pastry from scratch, or a ricotta and spinach roulade, which takes many stages to prepare. These fabulously delicious meals come at a price: time. For the rest of the week time is of the essence: I simply do not have enough of it, between the demands of work, ferrying children around, homework and the dreaded housework (I speak only for myself on this subject). So I need to know that I can beat the clock on the hypothetical takeaway meal or ready-made pizza from the freezer. I need to know that these options are not worth bothering with – and I do. I cannot therefore use 'not having enough time' as an excuse for poor-quality fall-back dinners such as fish and chips or 'the Chinese'.

I always start with the carbohydrate component of dinner. As you have learned by now, it forms the basis of any meal for your family. I can do rice, perfectly, in no more than ten minutes from walking through the front door. How? Preparation is my strategy. I boil a kettle of water as soon as I walk through the kitchen door. I also put on the oven if I plan to use it for this meal. Then I ask myself, 'Now, what will we have tonight? Will it be rice or potatoes or couscous or corn on the cob?', for instance. I put some basmati rice, as an example, in lots of boiling water and pop the saucepan on the hob. When it comes to the boil I place a lid firmly on and turn off the heat. In eight minutes, the rice is tender and then I drain it, place the lid firmly back on and it is ready to fluff up with a fork when I'm ready to serve it. I gave up on matching exact quantities of rice to water many years ago, as I know I will get distracted and it will burn! Now I use an egg-timer to measure the eight minutes and this is a foolproof method. When it comes to potatoes, I put the boiling water in the bottom of a steamer and place my pre-washed baby potatoes (skin and all) in the top of the steamer. These are also done in about eight to ten minutes. As for couscous, it takes three minutes in boiling water (correct measurement in this case) and corn on the cob can be cooked from frozen in the steamer, again in under ten minutes. As you might notice, you do not need only fresh ingredients here. Rice, pasta and couscous are dried, and therefore long-life. Potatoes can sit around for over a week before they start to lose their freshness. The corn on the cob I am most likely to use is the frozen, sweet variety that my kids love best. I actually find the 'fresh' ones can often be quite old and thus not so sweet. Stocking your store cupboard and freezer with such essentials is the only way to ensure the guaranteed ten-minute dinner I refer to here.

So that's the carbohydrate basis for the meal sorted. What next? Meat, fish or eggs – I tend not to do too many 'vegetarian meat alternatives'. Since for the most part I stay away from processed foods for my kids, I do not buy into Quorn or TVP (textured vegetable protein) or 'vegetarian burgers' and the likes. I might instead make a bean casserole or vegetable and bean curry, using whole foods yet again. While the beans, chickpeas, lentils, kidney or mixed beans might have come from a tin in my store cupboard (not since I was a young, free and single student have I soaked a pot of beans overnight and boiled it for three hours; I buy mine tinned), they are rinsed and drained of any preservatives (usually sulphites), and are good-quality, high-fibre, natural vegetarian alternatives to meat.

If it is chicken or white fish I want to cook I might simply add red pesto and place in the oven (no other labour required) or fry direct in the pan with a little olive oil (and a lid on top to speed up cooking time). If we are having steak I might quickly chop some onion, red pepper and garlic (this comes down to the frame of mind you are in, but it takes about three minutes in total) and add to some olive oil in a non-stick frying pan. I might add some mushrooms and as soon as they are cooked I take them off the pan and flash-fry the steak (i.e. cook it at high speed so that it is charred on the outside and juicy on the inside).

I cook eggs regularly, for reasons of health and speed. The egg contains a perfect source of protein, is cooked in three minutes and tastes great in many different guises. Scrambled eggs (whisked with a little milk, salt and pepper) cooked in a non-stick omelette pan in a little butter and olive oil over a low heat are fabulous, especially when slightly undercooked and runny. I do a complicated-sounding frittata in less than ten minutes. I simply chop some onion, garlic, pepper and tomatoes and fry them gently for two or so minutes in a little olive oil (the usual suspect!). I add the whisked eggs and let them set for a further three minutes over a gentle heat. I will have turned on the grill in readiness and finish the frittata by adding some feta or Parmesan to the top (depending on what is in the fridge; it could as easily be some left-over Cheddar) and placing it under the grill, where it bubbles up and becomes soufflé-like. As for the all-important vegetable component of the meal, I simply microwave, steam or sauté (fry in a little oil and possibly garlic) a nice colourful array of vegetables in under three minutes, while the frittata is under the grill.

As you can see, the speed of preparation relies almost entirely on having meat, fish, eggs or legumes (i.e. beans, lentils, chickpeas) readily available in a form (fresh, frozen or tinned) that you enjoy and that you know what to do with. Having a frozen steak in the freezer will be of little use to you unless you took it out that morning and placed it in the fridge to thaw out all day. Having frozen fish, however, is an absolute life-saver in my kitchen. Any fish can be cooked safely from frozen. White fish does need pesto or sun-dried tomato paste or olive oil or butter on it to make it tasty, while the beauty of a frozen oily fish is that it can be simply grilled (on tinfoil if you wish to save on the washing-up, which I always do!) and it is delicious in its own right. The really lazy version of this, which I do occasionally rely upon, is to take the frozen fish direct from the freezer and put it into the microwave (in an appropriate container) and zap. Salmon can be on the plate, steamed and delicious, within three minutes of being taken out of your freezer. To serve it I often drizzle over it a little sweet chilli sauce, or ketchup for the kids. I buy eggs every week: they are so convenient I rarely let myself run out.

What about the vegetable portion of the meal? Surely these must be served fresh to give your kids the maximum amount of nutrients per bite? Not necessarily. When you look at vegetables' nutrient levels you can find that the vegetables that sat on the supermarket shelf for a couple of days, then in your cupboard at home for a couple more, contain in general considerably lower levels of certain antioxidant nutrients and vitamins than those in your freezer. Frozen vegetables, if they have been frozen quickly after harvesting, can actually contain higher nutrient levels than those sitting in your kitchen. Try, for instance, thawing out an enormous handful of French beans in the microwave. Then fry them in a little olive oil and garlic (or garlic olive oil). My kids always laugh about this one: in France on holidays, they think me 'weird' for ordering salmon or a steak with 'haricots verts', cooked as I describe, instead of 'pommes frites'. The vegetable portion of the dinner does not need to be more complicated than this. Of course, salad takes no effort at all to assemble. Simply put out some cherry tomatoes in one bowl and lettuce, dressed with a little Caesar salad dressing, in another and the job is done. I often just microwave copious quantities of frozen peas to accompany a microwaved salmon darne as described above. While in this instance dinner might have taken no more than five minutes to assemble, when served with ketchup it is a real winner with kids. It beats sausages and chips any day, from a nutritional standpoint, and is a lot faster to produce.

Of course, you may need to build up a repertoire of quick meals, the type that I discuss here, over time. Change does not happen overnight, but practise a small repertoire of easy meals over the next month and I guarantee that your frame of mind will change to a 'Yes I can' approach to cooking. It shouldn't be too daunting to peel and chop an onion, when that's the only bit of hard labour involved in making dinner that night.

You might wonder about the fat content of the types of meal I have mentioned. Fat is one of the key components that make our foods taste good. As this book has explained, our kids need a regular intake of good-quality fat. So in the pea and salmon story, the fat comes from the oily fish; in the steak, chicken or fish example, the fat comes from the olive oil or pesto it was cooked in; for the curry or casserole the onions will have been fried in a couple of tablespoons of oil at the start of the process; and so it goes. All dishes benefit from the addition of a moderate amount of fat. There might also be a little more fat in the salad dressing you are using on the greens that day. We need not to be afraid of fat. Fat is good for us. Fat is essential to the health of our children.

Finally, have a strategy when you shop. I generally advise my clients to stay out of shops as much as they can. Every time we go to a supermarket to buy, say, just bread and milk, we tend to come out with a bag full of food we never planned to buy, with a big hole in our finances as a result. Shops are designed to sell you products you did not want before you set eyes on them. There is no such thing as a bargain when you think of your current focus, which is to limit excessive calorie intake by your family. Two packets of your favourite biscuits for the price of one is not a bargain, it is a disaster waiting to happen. They will eventually get eaten. This should be no surprise to you. Equally, two steaks for the price of one is no bargain if you are eating out tonight, you have a chicken ready for tomorrow evening's dinner and there is no room in the freezer to freeze the steak. It will have such a short shelf life when it is reduced in price that it will have gone off by the time you want to use it. So have a strategy around buying food that involves order and a list. Stock your freezer as well as your fridge and cupboards and you will never fall prey to the instant gratification – as demanded by your kids – of a takeaway meal.

Forward to a fun, fit future

Enjoy your food!

You are now in possession of some of the facts that I have learned from people I have worked with over the last sixteen years, from my research, and from my own personal experience of my family, past and present. The rules are so simple to follow. The results are outstanding. I have trialled this approach with my own kids over the last ten years and I can safely say that they know a lot more about nutritional balance and the language of good nutrition than I did up to the age of twenty-five. They are slim, fit, energetic kids, with as much interest in food and chocolate as any other kid, but they are familiar with the notion of moderation when it comes to the consumption of sweet 'treats'. In fact, they embody the French traditional approach to eating, which is that they eat whatever they wish, within reason, with a structured daily approach. They eat dessert, but they also eat salad. They go to McDonald's (very rarely), but they do not crave it. It exerts no pull on them, as it is not a forbidden food.

As a family, we eat in an old-fashioned way, by which I mean we sit at the table to eat; we have rigidly set mealtimes; and lots of the foods we eat are the stuff of good old-fashioned fare (with a modern twist, perhaps). We rarely eat processed foods. There are no pasta sauces in the cupboards; no soup or gravy mixes are used in cooking; ready meals or takeaways are consumed no more than a few times a year. In essence, we have gone back in time to how we ate in Ireland and Britain thirty years ago and to how many of the French, Italians and our other European neighbours still do today. We are not 'Americanised' in our eating habits; we hold the fork in our left hand and we put the knife in our right. We should endeavour never to shovel food into our mouths, forkful after forkful, in my opinion! This is something I have to stay on top of with my kids. In every American film they watch they see kids and adults alike shovel their food on to a fork and no other utensil is ever seen to be used. We need to do better than that. We need to slow down and first cut our food into bite-sized pieces with a knife, before eating it with a fork. We also need our children to chew their food properly before swallowing it and thus register better how much of it they have eaten.

> In essence, we have gone back in time to how we ate in Ireland and Britain thirty years ago and to how many of the French, Italians and our other European neighbours still do today.

Instant benefits

On top of savings in calorie consumption, I can
guarantee you huge savings in money on your weekly
shopping when you follow my approach; huge savings
on calories for the entire family, including your kids,
and huge health benefits from all the nutrients your
family are going to consume every day.

You now have cupboards full of nutritious fresh and
long-lasting tinned and packaged foods. You rely
mainly on whole foods when preparing meals and you
have become confident in both your own cooking
skills and in the fact that your kids will most likely eat
what you set down in front of them at mealtime. You
are no longer stuck in the rut of having pernickety kids
whose pickiness restricts their consumption of foods
to those bland and tasteless varieties that tend to be of
very limited nutritional value. Your kids now look for
tasty foods; they no longer rely solely on salt and sugar
for enjoyment. Your kids have an ordered approach to
eating, where chaos may once have reigned. You can sit
down, as a family for the most part, and eat a balanced
meal together, without complaints, without the
distraction of gadgets or the television and with
conversation, instead of what may have been conflict.
You can rely on your kids to control themselves when
at other people's houses, out and about with friends or
at a birthday party. You no longer use food as the sole

reward for good behaviour in your family. Your kids no longer badger you for an endless stream of treat foods (those with too high a proportion of sugar, fats and salt), especially when going to the movies or for a Saturday night in. You no longer rely on takeaway foods as the only alternative to cooking a time-consuming dinner. You save yourself a fortune in both money and calories by having a well-stocked freezer and fridge, from which you can produce a family-friendly and tasty meal in less than twenty-five minutes (about the minimum time it would take to get a takeaway pizza or Chinese meal delivered or collected), with only ten minutes of effort on your part. Your kids are now able to taste the subtle flavours of more simple foods (the baked potato has replaced the potato waffle) and can acknowledge how overly salty the processed equivalent is, on the rare occasions they are exposed to it. You certainly do not ban them from going to fast-food restaurants or birthday parties held at same; you would rather your children have a confident approach to food, not the neurotic one we might have ourselves!

Your child and you as a family have started to move more. You are not as lazy as you might once have been, and yes, I am sorry to use the word lazy, but there you have it; many of us have become lazy of late. You now go to the bother of getting them up and out at the weekend to the park with their roller-blades or simply on foot to buy the Sunday paper, instead of allowing them to flop about the place all day, like fish out of water, lounging on the sofa watching television and looking for their next sugar hit. You treat them to treats other than food. You do go to the cinema, but without the accompanying calorie load; you do go to the pub for lunch, after a family jaunt; you treat them to new funky clothes because their old ones are too big around the waistband (and they can be put away for when they are older).

Your kids are now falling back in line with what it is nature intended for them. They are getting fitter, faster, and are having more fun. They are not a miserable mix of laziness and sugar-poisoning: instead, they are invigorated, nutritionally sound and fit to take on the world. Lucky kids!

Their future will be brighter as a result. In the short term, they may sleep better and get up feeling more alive and happier. Cheery kids in the morning are definitely worth fighting for. They may perform better at school, with more interest and concentration due to increased nutrient levels (iron being an obvious example here) and with less of the sugar-high, sugar-low pendulum they might have suffered from in the past. They may feel more confident (as a result of some weight loss, perhaps) and thus more willing to take up new sports and interests. They may begin to shine like never before.

In the long term you will have set them up to have sound eating habits for life. When they reap the benefits in the short term they will believe more in what you are doing and your only job after that is to reinforce the messages they have now learned by continuing with a consistent approach to applying these rules. You are also doing your best to protect your kids from ill-health as they get older, and from an early death from some of our most common killers – cancer, heart disease and type 2 diabetes. There is no convincing a child of the long-term benefits of this approach, as they live only in the here and now, but you will rest easy knowing you are setting them up for life.

The recently coined phrase 'overweight and under-nourished' is often used when discussing the health of US children. They are the first generation expected not to outlive their parents, as a result of excessive eating, of eating foods high in calories and low in nutrients, and of being obese. You are now in possession of the tools needed to equip your kids to do exactly the opposite. Your kids can now get the most nutrients possible for fewer calories than they were previously consuming. In doing so, they also get to eat more food, more volume, more bulk; in short, more fruits and vegetables. This relates to eating whole foods, for the most part, with plenty of good-quality 'treats' and only occasional 'rubbish' foods.

I am putting a recap of the rules here so that you have on one page (feel free to cut it out!) everything you have learned from reading this book. Apply one of these rules and you will benefit your child's health for life; apply two or three of them and they are going to have a healthier future. Apply all ten rules and you will have educated and empowered your child to make great decisions about food, for life. Knowledge is power. Once they have learned the rules they cannot unlearn them. And one day they will thank you for it.

RULE 1:

I can say 'No' to food

RULE 2:

Eat only at the table

RULE 3:

Have they had their fruit and vegetables today?

RULE 4:

We do not need to buy organic foods

RULE 5:

If you can name it, you can consider it

RULE 6:

Say 'No' to passive consumption

RULE 7:

Eat only when you feel hungry

RULE 8:

Get moving!

RULE 9:

Just portion control it

RULE 10:

Have a strategy

Index

additives 104–5
  artificial sweeteners 109
advertising and marketing 27,
  130–1
aerobic fitness 178–80
alcohol 136
American Dietetic Association
  100–1
'Americanised' eating habits 224–5,
  229
antibiotics in meat 95–6
appetite 135
  during sickness 139, 184
apples 89
Atkins, Dr 50
Australia 51

baking with children 8, 195–8
bananas
  'banana jam' 160
  muffins recipe 87–8
  taste and freshness 85
berries 89–90
  frozen 86
birthday parties 193–4
blueberries 185
bowel problems 195
Brazil nuts 212
bread: brown bread recipe 159
breakfast: suggestions 66, 156
broccoli 53, 68, 71–2, 101
Brussels sprouts 53–4
butter 110–11, 190–2

cabbages 77–9
calorie intake
    alcohol and snacks 136
    carbohydrates 51
    children and 44, 143–4, 213
    fizzy drinks 125–6
    smoothies 140–1
    see also 'passive consumption'
carbohydrates 50–1, 109, 156–7, 215–16
    intake for children 213
carrots 53, 56, 67–8, 97
    carrot and coriander soup
        recipe 57–8
    carrot and seed mini-muffins
        recipe 120–1
    curry recipe 70–1
cereals (in a box) 138
chicken 95–6
    curry recipes 70–1, 75–6
    goujons recipe 92–3
    with red pesto recipe 148
chickpeas 76, 117, 217
chocolate 83, 118, 192
    calories 147
cholesterol 102, 111, 118, 189, 212
chores see jobs for children
Christmas 38–9, 135
citrus fruits 101–2
coleslaw 206
colour in food 66–8, 82, 185–6
constipation 195
cost of food 84, 192, 226
    see also shopping wisely
crisps 198
cucumber slices 53
curry recipes 70–1, 75–6
custard and stewed fruit recipe 65–6

Denmark: ban on trans fats 190
desserts 61–3, 163–4
diabetes (type 2) 22, 132
dieting 50–1, 144–6, 150–1
    fat-free 210–11
dinner
    'en famille' 35–40, 160–1, 224

plate visualising 163
suggestions 134, 161–4, 215–20
see also recipes

E.coli bacteria 80
eggs 212, 217–18
    frittata 218
emails and movement at work 175–6
exercise 10, 129–30, 165–82
    aerobic fitness 178–80
    definition of 170, 178
    gyms 178–9
    and the nobility 181–2
    play as exercise 111, 170–5, 179–80
    recommended 179–81

'fat pad' 22
fats 53, 110–11, 188–92, 206–7, 210–13,
    220–1
    olive oil 212
    spray oil 87
fibre 160
fish
    frozen 218–19
    goujons recipe 92–3
    oily 53, 102, 110, 212–13, 219
    with red pesto recipe 148
fizzy drinks 125–6, 131
flapjacks 196
France: approach to food 2–5, 198
free-range chickens 96
frittata 218
fruit and vegetables 49–76
    bioactive compounds 101–2
    colours 66–8, 82, 185–6
    enticing children 52–4, 60–4,
        66–9, 85–6, 89–90, 157–8
    frozen 219–20
    growing your own vegetable
        patch 79
    organic foods 46, 67–8, 77–97
    recommended consumption 51–3,
        73–4
    stewed fruit and custard recipe
        65–6

'functional' foods 100–10, 118, 121

garlic 102, 111
goujons recipe 92–3
grapes: frozen 60
green foods 65, 117
gyms 178–9

habits 68–9
    time to form 64
Hippocrates 99
hunger and overeating 43–4, 153–6
    recognising hunger 136–7
    scale of one to ten 43
hydrogenated fats 188–92

Japan
    eighty per cent full 43, 154
    functional foods 100–1
jobs for children 176–7
    accompanying adults 178

lamb 94–5
    tagine recipe 152–3
lunch: leisurely in France 3
lunchboxes 33–4
    baking for 196
    fruit and vegetables 53, 61, 63–4,
        68, 85, 157
    sandwiches 156–7
    yoghurt drinks 106

McDonald's and children 4–5, 224
margarine 188–92
mash recipe 149
meals
    prepared by children 197–200
    time for preparation 214–15
    for suggestions, see also
        breakfast; desserts; dinner;
        lunchboxes; recipes
meat 213, 216–17
    organic 94–6
medicine and food 99, 121
milk 96–7, 107, 160
    low-fat 156

'movers' and 'non-movers' 165–8
muffins recipe 87–8, 120–1

neutraceuticals 100, 102
New Zealand 38–9
'nine out of ten' rule 202–3
'no' 54
nobility and exercise 181–2
nutrients
    in fruit and vegetables 82–3
    nutrition supplements 72, 138
    see also 'functional' foods

oats 84, 102, 111
obesity 2–3
oils see fats
omega-3 fatty acids 102
orange foods 67–8, 117
organic foods 77–97
    carrots 56, 67–8
    meat 94–6
    nutrients 82–3, 97
'over-parenting' 169–70, 172–3
overeating and hunger 43–4, 153–6
'overweight and undernourished'
        generation 229

parenting see 'over-parenting';
        'public parenting'
'passive consumption' 108, 126,
        139–42
pedometer 175
pesto with chicken or fish recipe 148
'picky kids' 138, 183–5
picnics 205
pizzas 130–1, 133–4, 163
plant stanol esters (sterols) 111
plate visualising 163, 208
portion control 128–9, 207, 209
potatoes 7
    crisps suggestion 68
    magic mash recipe 149
    volcano potatoes 196–7
    wedges recipe 94
probiotics and prebiotics 103–8

protein intake 213
protein plans and diets 50–1
'public parenting' 80–1

recipes
    Baby Banana Muffins 87–8
    Cat-food Tagine 152–3
    Chicken or Fish with Red Pesto
        148
    Curry in a Hurry 75–6
    Cute Carrot and Seed Mini-
        Muffins 120–1
    Dummy's Brown Bread 159
    Five-minute Carrot and
        Coriander Soup 57–8
    Fun and Tasty Chicken or Fish
        Goujons 92–3
    Kid's Curry 70–1
    Magic Mash 149
    Potato Wedges 94
    Smooth Sweet Tomato and Basil
        Soup 59–60
    Stewed Blood Fruit and Custard
        65–6
    Three-minute Tomato Sauce
        113–14
recommended amounts
    of daily calories for children 143–4
    of exercise 179–81
    of footsteps per day 175
    fruit and vegetables 51–3
rice cakes 80–1
routine and planning 31–3, 201–2
    workplace routine 175–6

salads 220
sandwiches 156–8, 205–10
saturated fats 189
    see also fats
sauces: tomato sauce recipe 113–14
seasonal food 89
shopping wisely 84–6, 90, 214, 221–2
    shopping list 114–15, 116
sickness and appetite 139, 184
smoothies 139–41

snack foods 117–18, 123–42, 156–8
    bed-time 194
    fruit and vegetables 52–3, 60–1,
        63–4, 68, 85, 89–90, 157–8, 160
    nuts and seeds 117–18, 212–13
    organic carrot test 97
    trans fats and 190–1
    see also sweets and treats
soups 55–6
    carrot and coriander recipe 57–8
    tomato and basil recipe 59–60
sterols 111
sugar
    in the bloodstream 132–3
    fat-free products 211
    sugar-free products 109
    yoghurts 106–7, 119
    see also sweets and treats
Sundays
    clothes 25
    tablecloths 38–9
supplements see nutrients
sweet potatoes 68
sweets and treats 16, 44–5, 144–5
    desserts 61–3, 163–4
    saying 'no' 47–8
    survival instinct 56, 62

table
    dinner 'en famille' 35–40, 160–1,
        224
    'eat only at the table' 31–48, 160–1
    tablecloths 38–9
tagine recipe 152–3
teenagers: sleeping late 46–7
television
    as babysitter 171–2, 180–1
    eating in front of 45–6, 126–31
    as treat 176–7
terminology around weight 20–1
time preparing meals 214–21
tomatoes 101, 111
    tomato and basil soup recipe
        59–60
    tomato sauce recipe 113–14

trans fats 188–92
travelling and food 201–5
   sandwiches on the hoof 205–10
treats 16, 44–5, 144–5
Tupperware 204
turnips 67

United States 2, 8, 132
   American Dietetic Association
      100–1
   'Americanised' eating habits 224–5,
      229
   'overweight and undernourished'
      generation 229

vegetable patch 79
vegetables *see* fruit and vegetables
vegetarians: meat alternatives 76,
      216–17

vitamins *see* nutrients

waistband measurement 24–5
   'fat pad' 22
wedges: potato wedges recipe 94
weighing scales 15, 23–4
weight-loss 50–1, 167
wet-weather gear 177
whole foods 84, 89, 91, 110, 226
   ingredients list 104–5, 118–19
workplace routine 175–6
World Health Organisation (WHO)
   footsteps per day 175
   olive oil 212
   overweight children 13
   portions of fruit and vegetables
      51–3

yoghurts 100, 103–8, 110, 118–19